ATKINS DIET FOR BEGINNERS 2021

EASIER TO FOLLOW THAN KETO, PALEO, MEDITERRANEAN OR LOW-CALORIE DIET

CONTENTS

INTRODUCTION

This book contains proven steps and strategies on how to lose weight by following an easy Atkins Diet guide.

Put simply, the Atkins Diet is a very effective and easy to follow diet, one which gives you guaranteed, effective results. The Atkins Diet plan helps you learn and recognize healthy food habits which will change your outlook on dietary nutrition for life.

No calorie counting, no red or green days, and nothing too complicated. Recipes use common ingredients and are easy to follow.

If you have picked up this book, then you are no doubt very interested in following the Atkins Diet and you are probably familiar with some aspects of the plan. First of all, we will reiterate the diet's basics, how it works, how it differs from other popular diets, and how to follow the diet. We will then explain the phases and what you need to do in each one. After that, we will get onto the practical stuff: the meal plans for each phase and corresponding recipes for the delicious meals!

The aim of this book is to show you that the Atkins Diet gives you endless choices and freedom when it comes to delicious meals and snacks. You don't have to be a super chef to be able to follow this diet and you don't need to spend a fortune on expensive ingredients – many ingredients for this diet are already in your fridge, freezer, or kitchen cupboards.

Thanks again for purchasing this book. I hope you enjoy it and transform

your lives and health!

1

THE BASICS OF THE ATKINS DIET

The Atkins Diet is derived from a best-selling book written in 1972 by cardiologist, Dr. Robert Atkins. The Atkins Diet is what is generally referred to as a low-carb diet.

Although quite unpopular upon its first emergence due to increased fat intake, the Akins Diet has gained increased popularity over the last decade. In this chapter, we will cover what the Atkins Diet is, how it works, and how to use it to your advantage as a weight loss method.

WHY THE ATKINS DIET WORKS?

The Atkins Diet is a four-stage diet that focuses on losing weight by reducing carbohydrate consumption. This reduction in carbohydrate consumption results in more stable sugar levels in the body, as well as decreased hunger, fewer food cravings, and reduced fat storage.

So, how do these benefits come about from simply reducing carbohydrate consumption? The Atkins Diet capitalizes on the fact that the body is able to utilize two different types of food groups for energy – sugars (carbohydrates) and fats.

Most people are familiar with the concept of the body utilizing sugars for fuel. As the body breaks down carbohydrates, sugars are produced in the form of glucose. These sugars are then used to feed cells to provide the body with energy. The body prefers to feed on sugars first because they are easily accessible and broken down. When foods result in too much sugar being produced in the body, the excess sugar is stored as glycogen in the liver. However, when the liver can store no more glycogen, the sugar is stored as fat throughout the body.

What many people are not aware of is the fact that the body can also utilize fat for energy. When there is no easily accessible sugar (as found in carbohydrates) to break down for energy, the body will turn to fat for the needed energy. Breaking down fat will release stored sugars that can then be used for fuel. Breaking down the fat in your body for sugar will then result in weight loss as these fat cells are destroyed. This process of burning fat for energy is called "lipolysis." When lipolysis takes place and the existing stores of fat are burned, the body then releases something called ketones. By eating a diet that is low in carbohydrates, you are forcing your body into lipolysis. This process can be maintained by eating a diet that is high in fats as it tricks your body into thinking that the fats that you are consuming are part of the natural process of lipolysis.

BENEFITS OF THE ATKINS DIET

There are many benefits to following the Atkins Diet which will be highlighted in this chapter.

First and foremost, you will lose weight quickly on the Atkins Diet. As much of the obesity epidemic in this country is due to eating refined carbohydrates and sugar, by eliminating these things from your diet, you will start to lose weight almost immediately. You can lose up to 30 pounds in 30 days on the Atkins Diet which is why most people go on the Atkins Diet. They haven't been able to lose weight on any other system, but can with the Atkins plan.

But beyond weight loss, there are some significant health benefits to following this diet. First, several studies have shown that following the Atkins Diet can reduce the risk of some contributing factors for heart disease, including lowering blood pressure, lowering cholesterol and triglyceride levels, and decreasing inflammation in the body which has been shown to increase the chance of developing heart disease.

Second, losing weight can reduce the risk of some kinds of cancer. Studies have shown that people who have lost weight decrease their risk of colon and breast cancer, even in survivors who are at risk of recurrence.

Low-carb diets such as the Atkins Diet have been shown to reduce the risk of cognitive impairments, such as diseases like Alzheimer's. If you eat low-carb, you may be reducing your risk for dementia.

If you have diabetes, going low-carb can be good for you. Many different studies have verified that following a low-carb diet, such as the Atkins Diet can decrease the symptoms of diabetes, improve the problem of insulin resistance, and can help with different metabolic disorders.

Studies have shown that the risk of women developing Polycystic Ovary Syndrome (PCOS), which is an endocrine disorder that can affect women in their child-bearing years, can also be reduced by eating a low-carb diet. It has been shown that this disorder is associated with obesity and insulin resistance, both of which can effectively be reduced by following a low-carb diet.

Low-carb diets were also shown to improve the problem of daytime sleepiness in people who suffer from narcolepsy, a disorder where people uncontrollably fall asleep during the day.

As you can see, there are many benefits to following the Atkins Diet. If you suffer from any of these diseases, you could see some significant improvements in a variety of medical disorders in addition to losing weight by following a low-carb eating plan.

2

HOW IS THE ATKINS DIET BETTER THAN OTHER POPULAR DIETS?

KETO DIET

How does the Keto diet work? When it comes to the low-carb diets, the Atkins Diet started it all. However, at the moment the Keto diet is the most marketed low carb diet. The ketogenic diet is a very low-carb, high-fat diet that shares many similarities with the Atkins and other low-carb diets. It involves drastically reducing carbohydrate intake and replacing it with fat. This reduction in carbs puts your body into a metabolic state called ketosis. The goal of the ketogenic diet is to achieve ketosis when the body is metabolizing fat at a high rate for the body's energy supply.

What You Eat on the Keto Diet? The "classic" ketogenic diet - or keto diet - was developed to treat epilepsy. Traditionally, it's extremely strict and should be done only under medical supervision. Classic keto diets include very high levels of fat (75% of calories), low levels of protein (20% of calories) and extremely low levels carbohydrates (less than 5% of calories) and may also be calorie restricted. On the Keto diet, you'll probably need to keep carb intake under 50 grams per day of net carbs, ideally below 20 grams. You should base the majority of your Keto meals around these fatty foods: meat, fatty fish, eggs, butter and cream, unprocessed cheese, nuts and seeds, healthy oils, avocados and low-carb veggies (most green veggies, tomatoes, onions, peppers, etc.). On a ketogenic diet, you should eliminate these foods: sugary foods (soda, fruit juice, smoothies, cake, ice cream, candy, etc.), grains or starches (wheat-based products, rice, pasta, cereal, etc.), fruit (all fruit, except small portions of berries like strawberries), beans or legumes (peas, kidney beans, lentils, chickpeas, etc.), root vegetables and tubers (potatoes, sweet potatoes, carrots, parsnips, etc.), low-fat or diet products (highly processed and high in carbs), some condiments or sauces (contain sugar and unhealthy fat), unhealthy fats (processed vegetable oils, mayonnaise, etc.), alcohol (alcoholic beverages can throw you out of ketosis), and sugar-free diet foods (high in sugar alcohols, which can affect ketone levels in some cases).

How is Atkins better than Keto? A ketogenic diet, as well as Atkins Diet, restricts carbs. Besides weight loss, both diets may help control blood sugar levels and avoid processed foods with added sugars. However, Atkins is a better than a ketogenic diet. On Atkins, you get more food choices and eat a greater balance of macronutrients as carbs are not eliminated and protein is not restricted. This allows you to eat a variety of satisfying foods. Most importantly, the Atkins plan is easier to follow than Keto. A classic Keto diet is very strict and medical supervision is recommended. Atkins Diet Phase 1 can be aligned to a Keto diet. In Atkins Diet Phase 1, you can eat up to 20 g or carbs which will be about 80 calories from carbs. That is very restrictive and in the Atkins diet, you need to follow that for about 2 weeks (during only Phase 1) only. When following a Keto diet, you have to follow this restriction of carbs as long as you are doing Keto diet. Otherwise, you will cancel ketosis. This key difference makes it much easier to follow the Atkins diet.

On the Atkin plan, you start with a very-low, ketogenic-like intake and then gradually add carb sources such as vegetables and fruit back into your diet. To sum up, Keto is a very limiting diet — you're eating mostly sources of fat, plus a little protein, and some non-starchy veggies — so it's difficult to maintain and it's typically intended as a short-term diet, not a lifelong change. Moreover, you will find that the products required to follow the Keto diet will be much more expensive than products for Atkins. Finally, Atkins is more sustainable because Atkins let you enjoy more food choices when aiming for weight loss and more varied food choices when you reach your goal weight. Atkins is more convenient, less expensive and offers more variety, making it much more sustainable long term.

PALEO DIET

How does the Paleo diet work? Eat the same whole foods that our pre-agricultural, hunter-gatherer ancestors ate. Several studies suggest that this diet can lead to significant weight loss (without calorie counting) and major improvements in health.

What you will eat on the Paleo diet? Grass-fed meats, fish/seafood, fresh fruits, fresh vegetables, eggs, nuts/seeds, and healthy oils. Avoid cereal grains, legumes (including peanuts), dairy, refined sugar, potatoes, processed foods, overly salty foods, refined vegetable oils and candy/junk food/processed foods.

How is Atkins better than Paleo? Besides weight loss, both diets, Paleo and Atkins, may help control blood sugar levels and avoid processed foods with added sugars. However, the Paleo diet doesn't include enough protein; sometimes the Paleo diet encourages dieters to eat grass-fed meats, fish, and seafood, but does not enforce a set amount that users must adhere to. Just like Atkins, Paleo is naturally low in carbs, but because it's restrictive and eliminates entire food groups, it's harder to maintain. Most importantly, the Atkins Diet is easier to follow than the Paleo diet. The Paleo diet limits things such as processed foods, dairy, refined sugars, and grains which may be hard for users to adhere to. Paleo focuses solely on the quality of carbohydrates, but neglects recommending daily intake amounts. On Atkins, an individual focuses on both the quantity and quality of carbohydrate intake. Atkins allows some convenience products to help keep you on track, as well as legumes and dairy. Atkins is an easier low carb lifestyle to maintain because you have a wider variety of food to choose from. Depending on your individual carb tolerance, starchy vegetables, whole grains, and legumes may be consumed in moderation. Unlike Atkins, Paleo's one-size-fits-all approach does not allow you to discover your personal carbohydrate tolerance. Atkins is more convenient, less expensive and offers more variety, making it much more sustainable for long term.

MEDITERRANEAN DIET

How does the Mediterranean diet work? The Mediterranean diet is based on the traditional foods that people used to eat in countries such as Italy and Greece back in the 1960's. Researchers noted that these people were exceptionally healthy compared to Americans and had a low risk of many lifestyle diseases. The Mediterranean diet is touted as a heart-healthy, primarily plant-based diet inspired by the traditional foods of the Mediterranean region.

What you will eat on the Mediterranean diet? Mostly plant-based foods (fruits and vegetables), potatoes, whole grain bread, beans, nuts, and seeds. Small portions of yogurt, cheese, poultry, and eggs are included. Fish and seafood is recommended twice a week. Oils (not butter) and herbs/spices. Limit: Sweets and red meat. Avoid These Foods: added sugar (Soda, candies, ice cream, table sugar and many others), refined grains (white bread, pasta made with refined wheat), trans fats (found in margarine and various processed foods), refined oils (soybean oil, canola oil, cottonseed oil and others), processed meat (processed sausages, hot dogs, etc.) and highly processed foods (anything labeled "low-fat" or "diet" or which looks like it was made in a factory).

How is Atkins better than the Mediterranean? Besides weight loss, both diets may help control blood sugar levels and avoid processed foods with added sugars. The Mediterranean diet doesn't include enough protein; Mediterranean diets do not give guidance on protein intake, except to limit red meats. This diet promotes beans and other lean protein sources. Sometimes Mediterranean diets have some specific limitations and guidance on how many times per week to eat things like fish and seafood. This diet, more than other diets, may require freshly cooked food, which can be hard for people with limited time. As the Mediterranean diet is higher in carbs than a low carb approach like Atkins, you might not lose weight as easily. Both Atkins and the Mediterranean Diet may help with weight loss and prevention of heart attacks, stroke, and type-2 diabetes, but studies show that a low carb diet may be even more effective at weight loss as well as preventing these health conditions. The major difference is that carbs are higher on the Mediterranean. They can make up as much as 40% of your diet! Some people can't handle that many carbs and will not be able to lose weight. The Mediterranean diet can be challenging for those who are carbohydrate intolerant since they may be consuming more carbohydrates than their metabolism can handle. On Atkins, you will learn to identify your individual carbohydrate tolerance, get to a comfortable weight and learn to eat for life. On Atkins, you can lose even more weight by discovering your personal carb tolerance - in other words, how many carbs you can have to lose weight and feel your best. With more flexibility on Atkins, you are also able to eat a wider variety of proteins such as lamb, beef and pork. Atkins teaches you to eat right, not less — a balance of high fiber carbohydrates, healthy fats, and optimal proteins.

LOW-CALORIE DIET

How Low-calorie diet works? A low-calorie diet restricts how much food you eat. You lose weight because you are consuming fewer calories than you burn.

What you will eat on Low-calorie diet? Low-calorie foods: low fat, moderate protein, and high carb. Low carb meals consist of lean proteins, heart-healthy fats, colorful vegetables as well as fruits and whole grains in moderation.

How is Atkins better than a Low-Calorie diet? A low-calorie diet restricts the total amount of calories which can lead users to feel hungry and unsatisfied. Being hungry makes it more difficult to stick to the plan. If users try to fill up on high volume food to combat hunger, low-calorie dieters may need to prep large amounts of very-low-calorie produce (celery, leafy greens, etc.). The diet also may require meticulous tracking of calorie intake to be successful. Sometimes Low-calorie diets count calories, but don't give guidance on types of foods. Users that aren't actively trying to meet protein requirements may not meet their protein needs as they cut back on overall food intake. Low-calorie diets do not limit processed foods with added sugars which can cause spikes in blood sugar.

A low-calorie diet is difficult to maintain and very often you end up being hungry, which makes it tempting to overeat. With Atkins, you count Net Carbs, not calories and you choose from a variety of satisfying foods. This way of eating naturally keeps your hunger (and calories) in check, and your metabolism starts burning fat for fuel instead of carbs and sugar which is a more efficient way of losing weight. A low-calorie diet restricts how much food you eat in order to lose weight. Atkins knows the best approach to weight management is to eat right, not less. Atkins, a low carb eating approach, may reduce common trigger foods that cause weight gains – like bread or a bowl of pasta. With the Atkins Diet, you can lose more weight with a low carb eating approach than you would from restricting calories. And you will feel healthier and more satisfied!

BEFORE YOU BEGIN

ATKINS YOUR WAY

The Atkins Diet program consists of four different phases. Your individual goals will determine if you need to follow all 4 phases one after another or you will skip first phases. So, give yourself a minute to answer these questions:

- Do I want to maintain a healthy weight or to lose some pounds?
- How many pounds do I want to lose?
- Do I want to lose weight fast with most limiting diet?
- Do I want to lose weight slow with least limiting diet?
- What foods do I want to enjoy?

Here is a quick overview of the four phases including what you need to expect from each phase.

PHASE 1 – INDUCTION

The first phase of the diet program is undoubtedly the most limiting. You will probably find it the most challenging of the four phases especially if you are fond of eating high carb foods. The switch is rather difficult. While you are not required to eliminate carbohydrate foods from your diet completely, it is still advisable for you to keep it at a minimum.

Entering the Induction Phase, you must steer clear of high carb fruits and vegetables. Instead, you can eat low carb vegetables including pepper, mushrooms, alfalfa sprouts, and leafy green vegetables. Instead of carb loading, you are encouraged to eat more protein food sources such as meat, eggs, and chicken.

You are also advised to consume healthy fats that include olive oil. Cheeses like cheddar, mozzarella, and cream cheese are acceptable. You may use herbs and spices such as cilantro, basil, and dill among others.

While this phase is the toughest, it also offers the quickest path to weight loss. The Induction Phase goes on for a minimum of two weeks. You can continue on this phase until you are 15 pounds away from your weight goal.

PHASE 2 – ONGOING WEIGHT LOSS

The goal of the second phase of the Atkins diet program is to help you find your personal carb balance. Some of the foods that you were deprived of during the first phase are allowed in this one. In the second phase, you may add high carb vegetables, whole milk, yogurt, berries, nuts, seeds and other cheeses such as cottage cheese in your diet.

You have to stay on this phase until you are only 10 pounds away from your weight goal.

PHASE 3 – PRE-MAINTENANCE

This is the phase where you have to reintroduce more carbohydrate food sources. While doing so, you are also expected to reach your weight goal. The third phase allows you to include the following in your diet: whole grains, starchy vegetables, legumes, and additional fruits.

PHASE 4 – LIFETIME MAINTENANCE

By the time you reach this phase, you should already be at your ideal weight. While your goal for the first three phases is to lose weight, all that changes in this phase. Your goal at this point is to keep your weight in control. You should still be mindful of the way you consume carbohydrates. Abandon mindfulness and you are most likely to regain the weight that you have already lost. To make sure you do not over consume carbs, you are encouraged to monitor your weight regularly

There is no due date for this phase. If you want to maintain your shape, you must make a permanent change.

4

HOW TO DO ATKINS

PHASE 1 - THE INDUCTION PHASE

Induction is the term used to refer to the first two weeks of your Atkins plan. During this time, you are going to eat under 20 grams of net carbohydrates per day for two weeks. Net carbohydrates are calculated by deducting your fiber content from your carbohydrate content. This phase is designed to start your weight loss as your body turns to existing fat stores to gain energy rather than concentrating on using sugars from carbohydrates as energy. During this time, you will focus on eating plenty of protein, plenty of high-fat foods and low carbohydrate vegetables.

The Induction Phase can be repeated at the end of two weeks if you still desire to lose more weight before introducing some carbohydrates. If, however, you are beginning the Atkins diet with only a few pounds to lose, you can skip the induction phase and move straight to the balancing phase.

There are a few rules that regulate the Induction Phase of the Atkins diet:

- It is important to not skip meals and you should never go 6 hours or more without eating.
- Try to eat fiber-rich foods to reduce the feeling of being hungry. You
- can eat either three ample sized meals a day, or you can eat five smaller meals per day. During each meal, it is important that you eat a minimum of 4-6 oz. of lean proteins including pork, chicken, fish,

lamb, veal, shellfish, eggs, cheese, and low carb vegetables.
- Your carbs HAVE to be limited to 20 grams of net carbs daily and 12 to 15 grams of these net carbs should be from vegetables.
- Try to avoid eating out until you are comfortable with your Atkins values.
- When using fats, use 1 tbsp. of oils or a small part of the
- butter. Eat only 4 oz. of cheese daily if eating cheese (this does not include cottage cheese or ricotta.)
- Atkins Diet bars are available specifically for phase 1 of Atkins and make a great sweet tooth satisfier.
- Drink eight 8oz. servings of Atkins approved beverages per day – water is best.
- Ensure that you are taking a daily multi-vitamin without iron, as well as an omega-3 supplement.
- Always count your carbs. Don't guess when it comes to carbohydrate content because the carbohydrate value of different foods can be deceiving.

Commonly consumed foods during the first phase of Atkins are:

- All fish
- All poultry
- All shellfish (muscles and oysters in moderation)
- All meat (no sugar cured or meats with nitrates added)
- Eggs
- Low carb cheeses (bleu cheeses, cheddar, feta, mozzarella, Swiss, parmesan, and cream cheese)
- Low carb vegetables (celery, cucumber, fennel, mushrooms, iceberg lettuce, peppers, and romaine lettuce.) These are mostly "salad" type vegetables. Avoid starchy vegetables.
- Some medium carb vegetables (artichokes, asparagus, avocado, broccoli, kale, onion, pumpkin, and tomato)

Other Things You Need to Know About the Induction Phase

The recommended number of weeks to spend on the Induction Phase is two weeks at a minimum. However, some people may take longer while others may require less time. In fact, some people may not need to go through it at all. It essentially depends on how much weight you want to lose to attain your ideal weight goal.

If your goal is to lose 15 pounds or less, you can jump to the second phase and skip this one altogether. However, if you want to lose more than that, you have to stay on this phase until you are only 15 pounds away from your desired weight. If you want to lose weight fast, you can stay on this phase for three, four or even five weeks. Keep in mind that drastically cutting carbs in the early phase of the program can result in some side effects, including headache, dizziness, weakness, fatigue or constipation.

What does a normal menu on the Atkins Induction Phase look like?

Again, you must consume an average of 20 grams of net carbs a day during the first phase. Most people feel that their appetite goes down on the Atkins Diet. They tend to feel more than satisfied with 3 meals per day (sometimes only 2). However, if you feel hungry between meals, you will find recipes in Chapter 6 and here are a few quick healthy snacks: a hard-boiled egg or two, a piece of cheese, a piece of meat, a handful of nuts, some Greek yogurt, berries and whipped cream, leftovers. You will find a list of acceptable foods in this chapter. You can use this reference to design your diet menu. Just be mindful of the serving size and the corresponding net carbs. Here is a 7-day meal plan sample to give you an idea. You are free to play around with the order of the meals as they are not cast on stone.

PHASE 1 MEAL PLAN

Monday

Breakfast: Mexican-style Eggs on Canadian Bacon

Lunch: Shrimp Fried "Rice"

Dinner: Faux Mashed "Potatoes"

Tuesday

Breakfast: Deviled Eggs

Lunch: Poached Chicken

Dinner: Creamy Soup with Mini Turkey Meatballs

Wednesday

Breakfast: Tomato, Green Chili and Chorizo Frittata

Lunch: Good Noon Tuna Kebabs

Dinner: Spinach Cups

Thursday

Breakfast: Italian Squash Pie

Lunch: Salmon Croquettes

Dinner: Cheesy Kale and Tomato Chips

Friday

Breakfast: Warm Chicken Salad

Lunch: Brussels Sprouts with Bacon and Parmesan

Dinner: Buffalo Hot Wing Cauliflower

Saturday

Breakfast: Minute Almond Coconut Muffin

Lunch: Country Style Garden Pasta Salad

Dinner: Apple Stuffed Chicken Breast

Sunday

Breakfast: Good Morning Atkins Waffles

Lunch: Coco Loco Shrimp

Dinner: Almond Balls

FOODS YOU CAN ENJOY IN PHASE 1

- Fish, meat, poultry or tofu. Aim for 1-1,5 palm-sized (4-6 oz.) portion per meal
- Eggs (up to 3 a day)
- Salad leaves (6 oz. a day recommended)
- Vegetables (7–11 oz. a day recommended) except starchy
- ones Whole-milk products (cream, cheese, butter)
- Oils (extra virgin/virgin olive, coconut, flaxseed, grapeseed sesame, etc.),
- Avocados, olives, tomatoes
- Full fat mayonnaise
- Unsweetened soy or almond milk
- Water
- Coffee, tea (without added sugar)
- Soda water, diet fizzy drinks sweetened with non-caloric sweeteners, such as Diet Coke
- Sugar-free tonic water, carbonated water
- 2 tablespoons of lemon or lime juice a day (to jazz up your water or salad)
- Low carb sweeteners, up to 3 times a day (Splenda, sweet, stevia,

xylitol, etc.)

FOODS YOU SHOULD AVOID IN PHASE 1

- Fruit, fruit juice
- Caloric fizzy drinks/juice
- Bread, pasta, muffins, tortillas, crisps and any other food made with flour or other grain products, with the exception of low-carb products with 3g of net carbs or less
- Any foods made with added sugar of any sort, including but not limited to pastries, biscuits, cakes, and sweets
- Alcohol in any form
- Nuts and seeds, nut and seed butter, and nut flours or meals (except flax meal and coconut flour)
- Grains, even whole grains
- Kidney beans, chickpeas, lentils, and other pulses
- Starchy vegetables such as carrots, potatoes, sweet potatoes, and winter squash
- Dairy products other than cream, soured cream, single cream, and aged cheeses
- 'Low-fat' foods, which are usually higher in carbs
- •Diet' products, unless they specifically state 'low carbohydrate' and have no more than 3g of net carbs per
- serving 'Junk food' in any form,
- Products such as chewing gum, breath mints, cough syrups, and drops, or liquid vitamins, unless they're sweetened with sorbitol or xylitol; you can have up to three a day of those
- Sauces which contain added carbs such as BBQ, cocktail, ketchup, pasta sauces, etc.
- Processed meats (products that are breadcrumbed, battered or flour coated, that contain fillers or added sugars)
- Low-fat cheeses, 'diet' cheese, 'cheese products', whey cheese or any cheese flavored with fruit
- Cow's milk for now as its high in lactose (sugar)
- Any salad dressings apart from full-fat mayonnaise or olive oil as

they are often high in carbs
- Vitamin waters

PHASE 2 - THE BALANCING PHASE

The balancing phase of the Atkins Diet should be put in to place after the induction phase – or multiple induction phases depending upon your plan. You should begin your balancing phase when you are no less than 15 lbs. away from your goal weight. The purpose of this balancing phase is to begin introducing some carbohydrates back into your diet. These carbohydrates should be lower in carbohydrate content, things like small amounts of nuts and seeds, or nut-based flours. During this phase, you want to begin with around 25 grams of net carbs per day. Despite increasing your carbs, you want to make sure to slowly add new foods to your diet by just eating small amounts of these at a time. Adding small amounts of mid-range carbohydrates will allow you to track how many carbohydrates you can consume per day while still losing weight.

There are still a number of rules that go into this stage of Atkins:

- You are still going to count your daily net carb intake
- You are increasing your carb intake, beginning at 25 g net carbs daily. This means the ability to add higher carb foods to your diet.
- You are still going to eat at least the same amounts of proteins and fats as you were in phase 1
- You are still going to drink the same amount
- You are still going to continue to take the supplements/vitamins you took in Phase 1
- Make sure, unless you have specific health conditions, that you are consuming enough salt. A lack of salt can increase fatigue.

There are a number of food additions to this phase of Atkins:

- Nuts and seeds
- Higher carb content dairy – cottage cheese/yogurt

- Berries

If you notice you are beginning to gain weight or that your weight loss stalls in the second phase of your Atkins plan, drop back your net carb intake a little and continue from there.

Other Things You Need to Know About the Balancing Phase

Starting at 25 grams of net carbs, you can increase your carbohydrate consumption at a rate of 5 grams per week. Stop adding only once you have reached your personal carb balance. While drinking alcohol is not encouraged for the first 2 weeks while your body is switching to burning fat for energy, it is fine to have alcohol in moderation after this 'Induction' period. Alcohol can be consumed in small amounts following Atkins which is a significant difference between Atkins and other popular diets. Stick to dry wines with no added sugars and avoid high-carb drinks like beer. Other low carb choices are vodka & diet coke, gin & diet tonic or whiskey & water for instance.

What does a normal menu on the Atkins Balancing Phase look like?

With the list of additional acceptable foods in your diet, you should be able to come up with a more varied menu plan. To give you an idea, here is a sample menu plan for the Balancing Phase.

PHASE 2 MEAL PLAN

Monday

Breakfast: Cheesy Sausage and Egg Scramble

Lunch: Stir-Fried Steak with Asparagus

Dinner: Creamed Cabbage with Chilies and Ginger

Tuesday

Breakfast: The Great Gazpacho

Lunch: Veggie Tuna Salad

Dinner: Grandma's Rustic Cole Slaw with Walnuts

Wednesday

Breakfast: Breakfast Stuffed Pepper, Mexican Style

Lunch: Fantastic Potato Gnocchi

Dinner: The Best Homemade Tots

Thursday

Breakfast: Breakfast Yogurt with Almond Surprise

Lunch: Atkins Chicken Veggie Bowl

Dinner: Black Beans and Quinoa

Friday

Breakfast: Blackberry Smoothie

Lunch: Mover Muffins

Dinner: Asparagus Wrapped in Chili Spiced Bacon

Saturday

Breakfast: Low-Carb Cheese Bread Snack

Lunch: Coconut Pie

Dinner: Super Stacked Eggplants

Sunday

Breakfast: Smoked Sausage with Special Dip

Lunch: Sweet and Spicy Chicken

Dinner: Roasted Vegetables in Herbs

FOODS YOU CAN ENJOY IN PHASE 2

Now you can enjoy all the foods you had in Phase 1 and widen your menu by including additional low carb foods:

- Nuts and seeds (except chestnuts and salted nuts
- Low carb fruits (berries, cherries, cranberries, melon)
- A wider range of full-fat dairy products (cottage cheese, ricotta cheese, yogurt or Greek yogurt), but limit whole milk to 4 tablespoons
- Low carb pulses (black beans, black-eyed peas, broad beans, butter beans, chickpeas, edamame, haricot or navy beans, hummus, kidney beans, peas, pinto beans, soybeans)
- 2 fl. oz. lemon or lime juice
- 4 fl. oz. tomato juice or tomato juice cocktail

PHASE 3 – PRE-MAINTENANCE

The fine tuning phase is undertaken once you are very close to your weight loss goal – you should be at the stage where you have around 10 lbs. left to lose. During this phase, you will add more carbohydrates to your diet. The purpose of adding even more carbs to your diet is to slow down the weight loss process and find your carb threshold for maintaining your weight rather than losing it. Another big goal to this phase of the diet is to begin seeing this eating pattern as a lifestyle change, one which you will maintain in order to control your weight and health.

There are a few things that you are going to do during this third phase of the Atkins plan.

The last 10 lbs. of your excess weight are going to be lost slowly during this phase. You will do this by controlling carb intake as you get an understanding of what your maintenance carb intake level is. Your goal during this phase will be to lose ½ lb. per week as your body settles into your new lifestyle.

This phase of Atkins is going to allow you to increase your carb intake a little more so that you can test whether you can maintain your weight with more net carbs added to your diet daily. This differs from what you did in phase 2 as in that phase, you were still losing weight and finding your carb intake threshold level.

Increase your net carb intake by 10 grams of net carbs weekly during this phase. Keep in mind, however, that you are still working to lose your last 10 lbs. If you find that this additional carb intake is stalling your weight loss or is causing you to gain weight, drop your carb intake by 10 grams.

By increasing your carbs you are going to get the chance to add more foods to your diet. This also affords you the opportunity to find out if any specific foods cause weight gain or any health concerns.

Your carbohydrate balance is the number you are trying to find during Phase 3 of Atkins. This number is going to be the number of net carbs that you personally can eat each day in order to maintain your current weight after you have lost the last 10 lbs.

Other Things You Need to Know About the Pre-Maintenance Phase

Since you are drawing closer and closer to your desired weight goal, you may start to feel a little more comfortable. You need to bear in mind a couple of things during this phase of the program. Knowing what to expect can save you from frustration.

Atkins dieters usually experience cravings and that is more apparent during the Pre-Maintenance Phase. Prepare yourself for uncontrollable hunger. This may happen because of reintroducing foods to your diet. Do not forget about forbidden foods. Steer clear from them. It is also important to listen to your body signals. Give your body sufficient time to adjust before adding another food group back into your diet.

If some foods upset your body, eliminate them for the meantime. Avoid them for a couple of days. Once your condition improves and you feel like your body's ready to give it another shot then go ahead.

Weight loss plateau is also common so do not be surprised when it feels like you stopped losing when you are not yet on your desired weight. Losing weight may have happened quickly during Induction. However, this phase is meant to be slow and steady. Be patient. Wait it out to know how your body responds. If you really have stopped losing weight and you need to lose a pound or more, cut back 10 grams from your daily net carb allowance.

Rather than a weight loss plateau, some dieters stumble upon their net carb tolerance which is ideal for maintaining weight. Make the necessary adjustment and make sure to focus on your goal all the time.

PHASE 3 MEAL PLAN

Monday

Breakfast: Pear and Pecan Salad

Lunch: Spanish Vegetables with Cauliflower Mash

Dinner: Quick Baked Tofu with Moroccan Rub

Tuesday

Breakfast: Green Tea Infused Cantaloupe Soup

Lunch: Mexican Surprise

Dinner: Creamy Green Beans

Wednesday

Breakfast: Quick and Easy Seared Scallops

Lunch: Macaroni Salad with a Twist

Dinner: Red Grapefruit Salad

Thursday

Breakfast: Braised Short Ribs with Horseradish Sauce

Lunch: Turnips and Caviar Afternoon Snack

Dinner: Brisket with Mushrooms

Friday

Breakfast: Cowboy Breakfast Skillet

Lunch: Peachy Prosciutto Bites

Dinner: Blackened Atkins Salmon

Saturday

Breakfast: Cheese Baked Atkins Eggs

Lunch: Baked Catfish with Broccoli and Herb-Butter Blend

Dinner: Broccoli Florets with Lemon Butter Sauce

Sunday

Breakfast: Broccoli and Arugula Salad

Lunch: Acorn Squash with Spiced Applesauce and Maple Drizzle

Dinner: Atkins Bbq Chicken Supreme Pizza

FOODS TO ENJOY IN PHASE 3

Now you can enjoy all the foods you had in Phases 1 and 2 and widen your menu by including these additional low carb foods:

- Higher-carb fruits in small quantities, starting with one at a time and only once a day (apples, apricots, grapes, grapefruit, kiwi fruit, oranges, papayas, peaches or nectarines, pears, plums, pomegranates, watermelon)
- Starchy vegetables (beetroot, carrots, corn, artichokes, peas, parsnips, potatoes, turnips, winter squash, yams)
- Whole grains (barley, cornmeal, couscous, kasha, wholemeal flour, wheat berries, bulgur, cracked wheat, millet, oat bran and porridge oats, quinoa, brown, red, or wild rice)
- Whole milk (increase your daily intake to 4 fl oz.)

PHASE 4 - THE LIFETIME MAINTENANCE

Once you are in Phase 4 or the Maintenance Phase, you are doing what you should for the rest of your life. You will maintain your weight loss by developing your permanent way of living in this phase. If you start to gain weight, you can always cut back your total net carbs.

By the time you are in Phase 4, you have been gradually increasing your carb intake to find your optimal balance, you know what foods you should avoid because they cause cravings or hunger, you have learned to be aware of your hunger cues and how to deal with them before entering into a food crisis, you know which foods are good low carb substitutes for high-carb foods that you used to eat, and you are comfortable with following the Atkins Diet for the long haul.

There are no new acceptable foods for Phase 4. By this point in time, you have added all the foods that you are going to. You should be comfortable with eating foods from each of the 3 phases and you should have found which foods you can and cannot tolerate. And remember, if you start to gain a few pounds back, you can always cut back your net carbs by 10 grams until you lose it and can maintain your weight again.

How to remain in control of your weight?

This is not a phase you will eventually graduate from - unless you want to run the risk of regaining weight. Therefore, it is crucial to stick to your carb tolerance level. This refers to the number of daily grams of net carbs you can take without gaining additional weight. This is something you will discover from the Pre-Maintenance Phase.

You should also continue allotting around 12 to 15 grams of your daily net carb allowance to foundational vegetables. Continue consuming about 4 to 6 ounces of cooked protein for every meal. If your carb tolerance level allows you to have two servings of fruit per day, do so, but never go beyond two servings in one day.

Carbohydrates, fat, and protein are all essential for regulating the body's blood sugar response. This is why the Atkins Diet program does not completely ban carbs from your diet from the very start. Make sure that your diet has all three not only for successful weight management, but more importantly, for your health.

Continue to monitor your weight regularly. Never allow yourself to gain more than 5 pounds. Take immediate action before it comes to that. You can prevent further weight gain by adjusting your carb consumption. It is best to keep counting your carb intake.

Be careful about serving portions. Some foods such as cheese and nuts may trigger you to overeat. To make sure that does not happen, you have to keep measuring. Stick to the assigned portions. Eat nothing more.

Make it a habit to drink plenty of water. Continue to read labels. This is especially critical if you are adding new foods to your diet. As you add new foods, observe how each one affects your body especially when it comes to your cravings and appetite.

Make time for exercise. If you engage in physical activity, adjust your carb consumption accordingly. This is to give your body enough energy.

Finally, you have to know the difference between hunger and habit. When you are overwhelmed with a feeling of hunger, ask yourself whether you are physically or emotionally hungry. Eat for physical hunger and not for emotional hunger.

Of course, as we have said, by this point in time, Atkins should be a lifestyle. It is not a diet. You should know which foods are good for your long-term weight maintenance and which is not. By Phase 4, you know that life is better on Atkins.

In this phase, you can enjoy all the foods that are acceptable in all of the previous phases.

5

HOW TO STAY ON TRACK

HOW TO FIND THE MOTIVATION

How do people stay on track when roadblocks get in their way? Use these simple strategies for success.

When you first start on a diet, the first few weeks are normally great, in terms of staying on track and feeling motivated. After a few weeks, this motivation can lag, especially if results have slowed after the preliminary push.

So what strategies can you apply to get you re-motivated?

Re-assess your initial plan and goals

When you're all fired up to get started, you frequently feel like you can reach your goal in no time and frequently results occur very quickly at first and then slow to a steady beat. So, after a few weeks, it might be time to review and aim for smaller goals. So, if you want to lose 30 lbs. then break it down into 5 or 10 lbs. mini-goals. Your goals should be inspiring, but not so big that they seem impossible and you're unable to apt them into your lifestyle.

Stressing about your initial goal can de-motivate you, so take this period to re-adjust, re-assess and then get right back on track. If your goal isn't too far away then maybe taking a few moments to think through it again may be all you need to recharge your motivation.

Give yourself something tangible to motivate you

This can be entirely up to you – it could be as simple as hanging a particular item of clothing on your wardrobe door that you want to fit into, so you see it every morning. Or write a list of WHY you want to reach your goal – improve your health and manage weight. Read these reasons every day if need be. Even going on Pinterest and finding motivational mantras and pictures can be an easy way of pushing yourself again. Telling those you love about the reasons why you are following this healthier lifestyle may encourage them to join you or at least give you the backing you need.

Deal with negative thinking

Everybody has 'off' days and you might have times when you feel overwhelmed by the whole process. If you're having one of these days, then talk to a friend, read some motivational stories or flick through some low carb cookbooks to restart your interest and get creative juices flowing.

If you do give in to negative thinking, then just write this off and begin again on your health journey the next day. The key to success is dealing with negative thinking and getting right back on track, rather than letting it spiral out of control.

Take responsibility

You're in charge for your own actions so don't blame others if things do not go entirely according to plan. It's too easy to do this and you'll be more likely to lose sight of your goal if you take this easy road. If someone brings cakes or cookies into the office, don't blame them for the fact that you eat some. If you slip, then take responsibility, enjoy every bite and then move on and get back on track.

Have fun with it

Rather than thinking it's a drag and the fun is sucked out of life, look at your healthy lifestyle in a new light. You shouldn't be eating 'diety' rabbit food on Atkins anyway, so explore some delicious low carb recipes and have fun with food. Even if you don't enjoy making new recipes, try experimenting with different cuts of meat or trying vegetables you've never had earlier. You never know - you might find some new favorites and it can stop you craving your old high carb foods. For example, replacing potato chips with celeriac chips might be something that you enjoy.

EATING LOW CARB ON A BUDGET

Eating healthier doesn't have to be more expensive and these tips should help! It's not a secret that many of the sugary or junk-filled foods are often on sale in supermarkets. The shelves are filled with promotions on sugar-filled drinks, biscuits, and other processed foods. However, how much nutrients are you actually getting from these foods? Almost none! So surely this 'saving' is not actually an investment in your long term health. Changing your lifestyle now is going to define your health down the line and may even help you skip out on drugs for high blood pressure, diabetes and other metabolic conditions. I hope these tips will enable you to keep the cost down when eating a low carb diet:

- The great news is that Atkins encourages the eating of dietary fat and fattier cuts of meat are often the cheapest! So cuts like pork belly, 20% fat minced beef and chicken legs or thighs are significantly cheaper than pork chops, lean beef or skinless chicken breasts.
- Vegetables are a significant part of the Atkins Diet and they are very

frequently on sale in supermarkets. If so, purchase in bulk and freeze the vegetables that you don't use. Purchase a huge cauliflower when it's on sale, steam it all and then freeze the half you don't use. You can use the rest to make a cauli-pizza base, cauliflower cheese or add it to soups, stews or other dishes. This is great for vegetables and fruits that are seasonal too. Buy it in season and freeze it for when it's not available in your local store.

- Local markets are also a great way to eat inexpensively as they are often much cheaper than supermarkets, especially for meat, fish and fresh produce. Visit your local market, even if it's once a month, and stock up your kitchen on essentials.

- Shop around! As well as your local market, try doing some of your shopping at other stores. They have great deals that can be much cheaper than the larger supermarkets.

- Buy frozen. If the vegetables that you like are cheaper in their frozen form, then go ahead. Just check the label as, unbelievably, some vegetables may have added sugar!

- Purchase in bulk and portion your food into separate servings. For example, purchase a whole side of salmon and then split into 8 or so portions and freeze. Much, much cheaper than buying individual portions.

- Eggs are a super food and so inexpensive! So stock up on free range eggs and you'll be getting a great source of protein and other nutrients.

- If you cook up double the portion size of your dinner-time meal, then you'll have leftovers for lunch the next day which can save you cash. It's much better to have a serving of low carb curry for your lunch than a boring old sandwich!

- Don't feed the family any differently. Atkins friendly meals can be delicious for the whole family, but just skip the starchy side dish from your plate. For example, if you have pork belly with roasted veg, give yourself cheesy cauliflower instead of the mashed potatoes that you may serve to the rest of the family.

LOW CARB DINING OUT STRATEGIES

We have covered the foods you can and can't eat during the Atkins Diet and its different phases. However, even if you strictly adhere to those rules, things get much tougher when you go out, especially if you are heading for dinner with your friends. On the one hand, you shouldn't avoid socializing just because of your diet, and on the other, it might be tricky to order food that's in accordance with your new way of eating. However, there is a way to find something that's appropriate for the Atkins Diet in all restaurants.

Before we head to tips about specific cuisines, let's take a look at some general tips about restaurants:

- You are a customer – and the restaurant is in the business of serving you and trying to get you come back again and again. That is why you shouldn't be shy to ask specific information about the ingredients that are part of a dish. The waiters might not know everything, but ask them to find out. You don't have to explain yourself, but make sure to be polite to the waiters and be generous with a tip if you put them through a lot of trouble.
- Research the restaurant – most of them have their menus listed online, which is why you should take a look at their websites and see if they are offering low-carb dishes
- Don't believe the menu – yes, that dish might seem healthy, but does it come with a sauce full of additives and sugar? There is an overall effort from restaurants to move towards the healthier menus, but what exactly defines "healthy?" Make sure that you find out all ingredients that go into the dish that you are ordering.
- Salad can always be a good choice – as long as it is Greek or Italian, as the dressing will probably have an oil and vinegar base. The thing you need to focus on is choosing the dressing. If it doesn't seem like what you are looking for, feel free to pass.
- Simple dishes are also excellent choice – grilled, roasted, or broiled fish and meat are probably the safe way to go. Stews are something you don't want to choose when eating out because they probably have starchy vegetables as well as gravy.
- Portion control is crucial – some restaurants have rather big servings,

but there is no need to eat everything just because they served it like that. Make sure to ask that the leftovers are packed in a doggie bag.

You can eat low carb and still enjoy a meal at a restaurant or take away by following these tips. Even for experienced Atkins followers, dining out can be a minefield and often where many of us slip up and give into high carb food. However, you don't have to avoid eating out just because you're following Atkins. You can eat low carb quite simply even when you're out. Here is some basic advice on how to make the best choices, based on the most popular types of restaurants:

Chinese

The best choice would be a stir-fry such as chicken, beef, tofu or prawns; though check that the meat/fish isn't breaded. It's better to avoid sauce on your stir-fry as these will usually be loaded with sugar or cornstarch. Alternatively, get a sauce on the side so you can control how much you have as, naturally, you get way too much anyway! Obviously, pancakes, noodles, and rice are out so ask for extra veggies if required. For the main courses, you can get lots of vegetables and it tastes great mixed with the meat. Beef & mushrooms is a common dish as well and a fairly low carb choice.

Italian

Skip pasta, rice and pizza sections as they are all sky-high in carbs. There are other tasty options such as porchetta (pork belly), typically stuffed with garlic and Italian herbs. For a starter, antipasto is a great choice consisting of assorted meats, cheese & vegetables such as olives. Some main courses such as chicken or seafood are fine, but ensure they aren't breaded. Most 'fresh' tomato sauces don't have a lot of sugar if made true Italian-style; check with your waiter to see if the sauce contains added sugar. As a replacement for garlic bread, opt for a tasty salad such as rocket & goat's cheese, for instance.

Pub-Style

Most pub-style meals focus on a protein base such as chicken, beef or fish with a starchy side of chips or mash with a small portion of vegetables. Steak, fish, poultry or other seafood are all fine as long as not breaded or marinated in sugary sauces. As an alternative for the chips or another carby side, ask for extra veggies or more side salad. You can dress it up with butter on your veg or full-fat mayo or olive oil on your salad. Burgers and cheeseburgers are fine as long as you ditch the bun and have a salad as an alternative for chips. Chicken Caesar salad is a good choice as long as you ask for no croutons.

Indian

Avoid rice as a side when taking a curry; it tends to 'stodge' the meal anyway and dilute the taste of the fresh Indian spices used. Good choices include meat or fish tandooris which are marinated in yogurt or sometimes cream to tenderize the meat, but are then fired in a clay oven. Meat/chicken kebabs or lamb cuts are fine too and usually are just marinated in spices & oil. Avoid naan or chapatti bread and ask for veggie sides instead.

Thai

Similar to Chinese cuisine, Thai base their cuisine on noodles and rice. The main thing to avoid is fried rice, but you can always opt for sautéed mixed vegetables instead. Choose sautéed chicken, beef, and even shrimp or scallops. Avoid spring rolls or dumplings as well as Thai curry because it can contain potatoes. You should also get information on sauces and make sure that they are served on the side.

Mexican

Avoid, and I'll repeat, avoid salsa and chips. However, you can try guacamole which is avocado-based. A great substitute for chips is jicama sticks which you can combine with guacamole. You can also order enchiladas verdes as long as you make sure that there is no tortilla and the sauces are not thickened. The same goes for fajitas except that you should skip the beans. Grilled chicken wings and fish are better options than chimichangas.

French

French are true gourmets, which is why you have a vast selection of meals to try. You can't go wrong with the classics, such as French onion soup (make sure that it's without croutons) and Boeuf Bourguignon (simmered beef cubes with garlic and onions). Things that you should avoid include croquet monsieur (sandwich), veal Prince Orloff (it contains rice), and vichyssoise (soup). However, you should make sure to try bouillabaisse (fish stew) and coquilles St. Jacques (brilliant scallops). For dessert, try some incredible French cheeses.

These tips should have you prepared for eating out. Remember – just because you are on a diet doesn't mean that you should avoid hanging out with your friends and people close to you. What you need to do is make smart choices and have enough willpower to pass up on unhealthy dishes.

Remember, restaurants love repeat customers so don't hesitate to ask what's in a dish – say you have an allergy if you're uncomfortable! Checking the online menu before you go out is a good strategy too. This way you aren't attracted by your old favorites when you're handed the menu. You will have already made your selection and more easily stick to it.

It is quite easy to follow the Atkins Diet when eating out in most restaurants. In summary, get extra vegetables instead of bread, potatoes or rice, order a meal based on fatty meat or fatty fish, and get some extra sauce, butter or olive oil with your meal.

6

KEYS TO SUCCESS ON ATKINS

ATKINS CHALLENGES AND HOW TO DEAL WITH THEM

As with any diet, there are some things that you should be aware of when following the Atkins Diet. Once you are aware of them, you can deal with them effectively.

First, some people do find that they feel weak or lethargic in Phase 1 of the Atkins Diet. As has already been discussed, you can move to Phase 2 fairly quickly, as soon as two weeks after starting the diet. Once you enter Phase 2, you will lose weight a little more slowly, but the problems of tiredness and the feeling of deprivation will be less. If you choose to stay in Phase 1, make sure that you are getting your entire 20 grams of allotted net carbs. Doing less than this will have adverse effects on how you feel.

The Atkins Diet has multiple benefits and weight loss is usually the one that people love the most. Aside from that, it can contribute to your overall health in various ways. However, a low-carb nutrition plan is not necessarily a perfect fit for everyone. The majority of people do experience an improvement in health and a better quality of life, but there are some risks and concerns you should be aware of.

The main thing you need to make sure is that any diet you are on is not too difficult for you. If you feel that it is overwhelming for your mind, the chances are that it's also too much for your body. If you think the Atkins Diet is restricting you too much, you might end up gaining even more weight if you discontinue this nutrition plan (after being on it for a significant amount of time of course; a couple of weeks can't do much harm).

A variety of factors can affect how you will feel about being on the Atkins Diet – your age, gender, genetics, body weight, as well as activity level and your medical history. Depending on these factors, the diet might be incredibly easy or extremely hard. Some of the risks and possible side effects of the Atkins Diet include:

- Fatigue and lethargy – it usually only happens until you get used to the new nutrition plan. After the initial couple of weeks, you should feel an increase in energy.
- Digestive issues, such as constipation – low carb diets may cause constipation in some people. This is because you cut out most of the fiber that your body is used to and fiber is one of the things that help keep your bowels moving. To avoid constipation, there are a couple of things you can do. First, make sure to get 12 to 15 grams of net carbs in the foundation's vegetables that are listed in Phase 1. Those vegetables contain a great deal of fiber and will help keep things moving along well. Second, make sure that you get enough water. If you are dehydrated, you have a much greater chance of developing constipation. Getting at least 64 ounces of water or more will make sure that things keep moving.
- Trouble sleeping – also happens only in the initial phase of the
- diet. Trouble exercising, which is directly related to feeling
- tired or weak. Bad or weird breath – Being in a state of ketosis can cause bad breath caused by your body getting rid of acetone. Your breath (and sweat) may smell like nail polish remover, but that's just a sign that the diet works! However, you might need to have breath freshener by your side.

Before you start the Atkins Diet, it might be a good idea to consult with your doctor. If you have a health condition you are aware of, it strongly advised to do so. If you are pregnant, breastfeeding, or you are an older adult, the consultation should be a must.

The Induction Flu

The starting phase of the Atkins Diet is also the hardest one. It does require you to make a giant leap when it comes to nutritional change which is why it may come with some side effects. A significant percentage of the Atkins Diet users complained that they suffered from what's called "the induction flu" during the initial phase of their diet.

The induction flu occurs because your body is adjusting to becoming a fat burning machine. The symptoms include fatigue, lethargy, nausea, headaches, and confusion. These symptoms appear during the first week of the Atkins Diet (days 2 to 5 are the most critical).

The good news is that there is nothing to worry about!

The important thing to know is that these symptoms also go away by themselves. However, considering that the induction flu is caused by one of two things – dehydration and salt deficiency, there are also ways to fight it. First of all, you want to make sure that you get enough salt and water into your body. If you do experience some of the symptoms, the chances are that you can get better in less than an hour if you drink salty water (you can try broth or bouillon as alternatives).

One of the drawbacks that a lot of people complain about is that they do not feel that there is enough variety on this diet. Of course, it depends on your point of view. If you are a good cook, there are thousands of recipes out there that you can use during the various phases of this diet. When you have so many recipes to choose from, the possibilities are endless. In addition, as you move through the phases, your food options increase. Most people do find Phase 1 a struggle, but it becomes less so as they start to see the weight melt off and s they transition to higher phases where they can eat an increasingly wider variety of foods. Included in this book are recipes for each of the four phases for breakfast, lunch, dinner, and dessert. Once you have tried these foods, you can search the internet for additional recipes. The options are really endless.

LEARN FROM OTHERS: MISTAKES TO AVOID

During the more than 40 years of its existence, millions of people have tried the Atkins Diet. By learning from their experience it is possible to avoid common pitfalls. If you get familiar with the traps that might be waiting for you, there is a good chance that you will avoid them. Let's take a look at where people usually make mistakes once they start the Atkins Diet:

Not Eating Regularly

In the previous chapters, we mentioned that you should have three regular meals per day or break them into 4 or 5 smaller ones. That's the eating pattern that you need to stick to if you want the diet to work.

Another thing to make sure of is that the time that passes between two meals is as equal as possible. Important: Do not to let yourself spend 6 hours without eating (except when you are sleeping at night). Eating regularly will help you fight hunger and other cravings.

Not Eating Salty Food

Salt is essential in the Atkins Diet and there is a reason why a significant majority of recipes lists salt among the ingredients. Reducing your insulin levels leads to your body releasing water and sodium through urination. Sodium is a critical electrolyte, and you cannot afford to lose too much of it. A great number of side-effects related to the Atkins Diet are caused by the lack of salt which is the best source of sodium. There is no reason to steer clear of salty food when it should be encouraged.

Not Eating Enough Fats

The point of the Atkins Diet is to make the transition from burning carbs as fuel to burning fat. However, to make sure you do this properly, you need to take in adequate fats. The only thing to keep in mind is that you need to be careful with the selection of fats and choose only the healthy ones.

Not Finding Time to Relax

Modern life includes many stressors. Stressors also lead to adrenaline and glucose being released into your bloodstream. This affects your body's ability to burn fat as a fuel and therefore influences your diet progress.

Make sure to find time to relax whenever you are able and make an effort to manage stressors effectively. In addition, a good night sleep is vital because not getting enough sleep can lead to an increased appetite.

Not Acknowledging Your Success

Being on a diet is hard – being on the Atkins Diet requires significant effort on your part. The good news is that the effort is quickly followed by the results. Whenever you feel like you made a small victory, take the time to acknowledge it. It doesn't matter how big the win is – did you just successfully manage dealing with sugar craving or did you just lost another pound? Bravo, you deserve applause, even if it's from yourself!

NUTRITIONAL SUPPLEMENTS

The dieting mode (Atkins) is an excellent way to lose weight efficiently, quickly, and without having hunger cravings. However, certain critics believe that you can't achieve balanced nutrition while you are on the Atkins Diet. We do have to consider this issue seriously because Atkins does make you avoid some foods rich in vitamins, such as certain grains and fruits. On the other hand, you are eating many healthy fats, amino acids, and proteins, so it isn't that you are not taking in nutrients and vitamins.

So, Do I Need Supplements?

The short answer is – yes. Believe it or not, Dr. Atkins himself recommended them in the original book. He might have found a way for you to lose pounds quickly, but he also had your health as a top priority. We will get to his formula for the nutritional supplements you need a bit later. Let's just take a look at a couple of benefits that taking them will bring you:

- You will ensure that you will get the full spectrum of nutrients that your body needs daily.
- They will contribute to the fat-burning within your body and help you get rid of those added pounds even more quickly.
- They can prevent some of the common problems that occur during the diet and they can help to avoid hunger from occurring.

Which Supplements Do I Need?

When it comes to Phase 1, it is a great idea is to take a multivitamin. The Induction Phase doesn't last long enough for your body to suffer from any deficiencies caused by the limited food list, but the nutritional supplements will help you fight food cravings and boost your energy and mood. The multivitamins might be the key to getting through the Induction Phase.

Other supplements can include green tea extract and chromium for fighting sugar cravings, as well as potassium, magnesium, and L-carnitine. Make sure to check the label of your multivitamin supplement because some of these nutrients might be included.

Once you reach Phase 2, there will be somewhat less need to add supplements to your diet. However, you might still experience sugar cravings or tiredness, so make sure to keep taking a complex of vitamins and the other supplements mentioned.

If you experience constipation, think about taking an additional fiber supplement, such as psyllium husk or flax seeds. You can use them in your meals (sprinkle them on top of what you are eating) or buy some tablets. You can also use Omega 3, 6, 9 oil capsules because they might improve your overall health, protect your heart, and enhance blood flow.

Finally, in the last phase, you are allowed to eat most foods, and your system will have adapted to being on a low-carb diet. There is no particular need to take supplements in the Maintenance Phase except if you experience issues such as fatigue, constipation, or hunger and sugar cravings.

The Atkins Supplement Formula

Dr. Atkins devised a particular Basic #3 formula to complement the diet he tailored. The product contained a variety of almost minerals and vitamins, and some of them, such as Vitamin C and E, were in a larger quantity than their recommended daily value. However, the Atkins Basic #3 formula is not in production anymore because Atkins' company changed its marketing strategies after his death. Below you will see the list of supplements that the creator of the diet recommended to include. You will notice that it is not much different from the supplements listed in this chapter:

- Calcium, potassium, magnesium – to help you deal with "induction flu."
- Chromium – to normalize blood sugar levels and lower cholesterol levels – no more than 1000 mg a day.
- Multivitamin formula – must contain high levels of Vitamins B and C – it will improve levels of energy, deal with sugar and hunger cravings, and ensure that your body uses the nutrients it gets.
- Essential fatty acids – fish oil, borage oil, or flaxseed oil. You can also use any Omega-3 capsules. Essential fatty acids will to protect your arteries and improve heart health.
- Fiber – to prevent constipation and contribute to healthy
- digestion. Co-Enzyme Q10 and L-Carnitine – assists in fat-burning and getting the body into ketosis quickly.

TIPS ON CONTINUED SUCCESS ON THE ATKINS DIET

As you begin your journey to a healthier lifestyle, you are going to come up against adversity. Whether it's cravings, cookies, or a nice, hot slice of pizza, you will struggle in the beginning. If it were easy, then the world would not be facing an obesity pandemic. The problem with giving in is that failure has a snowball effect. One candy bar is not going to thwart your overall goals, but continuous cheating will. Carbs are a rollercoaster ride of ups and downs. You will have cravings in the beginning, but as long as you stick with your plan, those cravings will go away.

However, an individual's perspective on the diet that can make the difference in whether the journey is a success or not. People often focus on meals themselves and forget that diet, especially an eating plan like the Atkins Diet, is a lifestyle change.

That's not the mistake you want to make which is why you should take a look at these tips that will make embarking on the Atkins Diet journey easier:

Never Stop Tracking Carbs

You should never stop counting carbs, even when you are on Phase 4 of the Atkins Diet. This is where keeping a food journal really comes in handy. You should always keep your diet under 100 grams of carbs. While going over one day is not going to hurt, you might quickly find yourself breaking that 100 -gram mark every day if you're not keeping track. Study after study has found that people who track what they eat have greater success with a weight loss plan (any weight loss plan) than those who do not.

Watch your calorie counts.

You do not have to count calories on the Atkins Diet. Nevertheless, it is important that you do not overeat either. If you follow Atkins, but eat 3,000 calories a day, your body will have fats to burn for fuel from your food instead of your stored fat which will hinder your weight loss. Most women should eat between 1500 and 1800 calories and most men between 1800 and 2200 calories. Your portions should be sensible. Restaurant size portions are often too big. Eating sensible portions will help you maintain your weight loss gains.

Be Sensible about Portion Sizes

You need to be sensible without obsessing about portion sizes. There are ways to do this with very little effort. For instance, replace your standard plates with smaller ones. Always wait at least 15 minutes before going back for seconds. In most cases, you'll find that you won't even want seconds after 15 minutes. You should be tracking your calories to make sure you're getting enough. Believe it or not, I've known people whose appetite became so suppressed that they ended up not eating enough calories. This resulted in a significant metabolic loss.

Never Allow Yourself to go Hungry

I know! A diet where you are told never to go hungry is not how we've been raised, but the truth is that you should always eat when you're hungry. What's important is that you eat healthily. Have snacks readily available. A small amount of nuts or seeds, or even a small piece of fruit, is an excellent snack choice.

Protein Should Be Included with Every Meal

Always include protein with every meal. You should eat at least 4 ounces with every major meal. Eggs or meat work fine. Protein has a way of filling you up longer. It takes longer to digest than simple carbs, so, when you get enough protein, you will feel fuller longer, which helps you stick to the plan (especially in the Induction Phase).

Savor Fatty Foods

Avocados are loaded with fat and they are on the list of the healthiest foods on the planet. Fat is the key to being successful on the Atkins Diet. Just be sure that the majority of your fats are healthy ones. Trans fat is the only fat you should avoid altogether since it's manufactured in processed meals. Every other fat can be a healthy part of the Atkins Diet. Make sure to get enough fat to feel full. It can be difficult to have most of your diet be primarily fats and proteins because eating fat has received a bad rap. However, eating fat will help you control your carb intake and the fats that are recommended in the Atkins Diet are good for you! Eating processed foods with a lot of fat is not necessarily a good thing, but eating fats from vegetable oils, olive oils, and lean meats are important. You should make sure that you feel full after eating, but just don't go overboard.

Avoid Added Sugar

Even though you can consume 100 grams of carbs once you reach the pinnacle of your Atkins Diet journey, you should always stay away from any foods that contain added sugar. For instance, sodas should be permanently given up. You can indulge in the occasional diet soda as long as you don't overdo it. You should never exceed two diet drinks in a day. Also, remember that artificial sweeteners will lead to sugar cravings, so it's best to stay away from them most of the time. Stick to foods that contain natural sugar such as recommended fruits. Check all your foods for hidden carbs, especially if you are eating processed foods. Many things have sugars added for flavor, especially condiments such as ketchup, salad dressings, and others. Make sure you are aware of all these hidden carbs in your foods. Use low-carb foods (and still read the label) and stay within your net carb count.

Eat Plenty of Vegetables

Once you get to Phase 4 of the Atkins Diet, you should be consuming at least 15 grams of carbohydrates per day in the form of vegetables. You will be meeting your daily goal of vegetables while getting plenty of fiber. I find that the majority of my meals are vegetable based with added fat and a small portion of protein. You can choose meatier options as long as you're getting your 15 grams of carbs from vegetables.

Eat Enough Salt

Make sure to keep salt in your diet. As your body transitions from carb burning for energy to fat burning, if you do not get enough salt, you may suffer from headaches, lightheadedness, cramps, or a feeling of weakness or lethargy. By making sure that your sodium intake is adequate, you should be able to avert these symptoms as your body adapts to the new way of eating.

You Can Still Eat Out

Unlike other dieting programs, you can eat out while following the Atkins Diet since it's so flexible. Just pay attention to the menu and replace unhealthy foods with healthier choices. It doesn't take long to learn which foods you can eat and which ones you should avoid. While I usually encourage my clients to avoid fast food, you can occasionally indulge as long as you stick to the low-carb section of the menu.

Take Supplements

Supplements are an amazing way to enhance any diet because we sometimes lack certain nutrients. A multivitamin will fill in the gaps. You have to be sure that you are taking them in conjunction with a healthy diet, not in place of it. Some people will take supplements so that they can make unhealthy choices without guilt. I don't care what they claim; you cannot lose weight unless you clean up your eating habits. No amount of supplements will change that fact!

Measure Your Success

Track your successes so that you have a motivational tool right in front of you! Keep pictures of yourself through the entire process so you can visually see the changes. You can even measure your waist every couple of weeks so that you have another reference point to motivate you.

Set the Desired Objectives

For most people, their goal is the number of pounds they want to lose or the ideal weight they want to reach. Perhaps you just want to make changes your current eating habits because they are deeply unhealthy. Whatever your motivation is, make sure to note the desired goals and remind yourself of them often. You can even spread little notes around your home so that you will read them each time you pass by them. Willpower and motivation will ensure success on the Atkins Diet.

Feel Free to Discover New Recipes

Yes, you might be restricted when it comes to the variety of food (at least in the initial phase), but there are many recipes that can be utilized. Head online or purchase a book of recipes that fit with a low-carb diet. Make sure that you try out a variety of recipes.

Find a Way to Motivate Yourself

Motivation is what should keep you going over the long haul. You need to think about what will make being on a diet more fun and less challenging. You can ask a couple of friends to join you and start the Atkins Diet with you. That way you can motivate and help each other push through the hard moments and cravings you will undoubtedly have at some point. Another way is to tell your friends and family that you are starting the diet and that you need their support. They should try to ask you how is it going as often and possible and try to motivate you to continue.

Finally, an excellent way to motivate yourself is to keep track of your progress. Make sure to note down your weight on the day you start the diet. Next, use a scale and write the exact number of pounds after several days (three or four). If you've stuck to the Atkins Diet style, you will notice progress. A small one, but hey – it's still progress. Continue using a scale every several days, and it should give you a boost of motivation. Alternatively, you can also look at yourself in the mirror and see how your arms, waist, and butt, are progressing. The important thing is to acknowledge the success you have been making.

Drink Enough Water

It is globally advised that one should drink eight glasses of water, but if you feel like drinking more – do it. Staying hydrated is crucial for low-carb diets. You will also probably have increased urination during the first few days, which is another reason why you should compensate with extra water. Most people go through life dehydrated and don't even know it. It is important to note that when you are dehydrated, it may feel like hunger. This is one reason some people eat too much. Instead of eating when you experience feelings of hunger, start with a glass of water. The color of your urine indicates whether or not you are dehydrated. You want to make sure that your urine is light yellow or clear. If your urine is dark, it means that you aren't getting enough liquid.

Plan Your Foods

Another tip that many people have found especially helpful is to plan your meals ahead of time. When you know what you are going to eat, it will be easier to avoid trips to the vending machine when a 3 p.m. food craving strikes. When you have a sensible snack ready for you to eat, you won't be tempted by junk food. If you have planned your food, you will be ready to face the day without fear of getting hungry.

Don't Look at Other People

Avoiding comparisons to others is a lifestyle rule will come in handy regardless of you are on the Atkins Diet or not. You are a unique human being and there is no need to compare yourself to others. That being said, each person works differently which means that some of us will lose weight more quickly and some of us will lose it at a steadier pace. However, who cares if your neighbor lost 35 pounds if you lost 'only' 20?

Learn to be satisfied with yourself and the progress you have been making. If you think that there is room for improvement in your diet, make the needed adjustment. However, if you are satisfied with your pace, make sure to acknowledge that.

Exercise

Regardless of the diet, physical activity and working out can contribute to your overall health and help you with losing weight. You might suffer from fatigue during the first couple of weeks which is why it is a good idea to take a break from exercising during that period. However, as soon as you have enough energy for exercise, get moving – go for a walk or a swim and head to the gym for training. If you include exercise is your daily routine, you will be much more likely to achieve long-term success.

Stay Motivated to Live a Healthier Life

We all have off days where we fall short and ultimately fail. The key to long-term success is to stay motivated. Setbacks happen. They are not what define our successes or failures, but the moment you lose motivation, you have started down the path of failure. This chapter will walk you through several tips that you can follow to help you stay motivated so that all of your hard work is in vain.

Don't Try Too Hard

One of the keys to long-term success is to keep things as simple as possible. When we try too hard and overcomplicate things, we lose motivation. It becomes confusing and can frustrate us.

If you feel like your motivation is slipping, then maybe you need to take a few days off from exercising. Or maybe you need to give yourself some kind of reward. The more an individual takes control of what motivates them, the more successful they can be in this area. If you put the right plan in place and keep it as simple as possible, then everything else will usually flow naturally. There is no need to overcomplicate anything.

Never Stop Learning About Yourself

Do you need to get the fastest dose of inspiration possible for weight loss? Then learn more about yourself. It is by far the most motivational thing you can do. By fully understanding ourselves, we also understand exactly why we are trying to lose weight in the first place. So when you start to feel the grind, ask yourself these questions:

If I give up now, how will I feel six months from now?

If I give up now, how will it affect my health?

If I give up now, how will my family be affected?

Be Realistic

Don't pin posters of super-thin models on your wall as a form of motivation because it will have the opposite effect. A significant number of studies have been done regarding this and the results are consistent. The problem with using thin models as inspiration is that most of us have very little chance of getting into that kind of shape. A lot of the time, these people are on super strict diets or they have time to exercise for hours a day. This is not an accurate representation of what most people can achieve.

Rather than aspiring to look like them, learn more about yourself and set goals that will improve your life. Post pictures of your progress. Pin up posters of inspirational quotes use daily affirmations as motivation. With the many options available, there is little reason to compare oneself to a model.

Focus on Specific Feelings

Sometimes we can become obsessed with an arbitrary number on a scale. It becomes a point of frustration and will cause us to lose motivation. That's why I told you to base your goals around processes rather than a number. Focus on your mood after you have eaten a healthy meal. Consider how much energy you have after an amazing workout. Weight loss motivation is not found on a scale; it's found in the way losing weight makes you feel. For instance, if you focus on how much better you feel after eating a healthy meal, then it reinforces just how positive a change you have made. This will increase your motivation.

Lay Out a Plan

All successful ventures start with a well-defined plan. This section will describe every step that must be taken to make your weight loss plan successful and a way of measuring your success. You should treat your health goals as you would a business plan. If you were trying to start a project for a client, then you would not go in blind. You would have a well-laid-out plan of action. We already know how to lay out a plan, but I want you to understand that you must follow through with it if you want to stay motivated through the long term.

Start Acting Healthier

The way we act ultimately shapes what we believe, so you should start acting as if you are leading a healthier life as soon as you begin the Atkins Diet. Do not wait until you "lose weight" to follow your ambitions. Start right away! Starting on the Atkins Diet is a new way of life. You need to treat it as such. Why would you put off your new and improved lifestyle until you achieve an arbitrary number on a scale?

Hang Inspiration Near the Mirror

Are you trying to lose weight before summer so you can fit into that new swimsuit? Then try hanging it near the mirror so that it can serve as a daily inspiration. Visualize yourself wearing it so that you are motivated to keep moving forward. Since you already own the item, this is not some unrealistic goal that you have set for yourself. It's very achievable and it will motivate you to keep pushing yourself.

Imagine Your Life if You Fail

Sure, envisioning yourself wearing that new swimsuit is quite motivational, but sometimes it can be just as motivational to envision your life if you were to fail. Ask yourself, "What will my life be like in five years if I do not stick to this plan?"

Sometimes fear can be the most powerful motivational tool at our disposal. Imagine how bad it could potentially be if you're still overweight five years from now. You'll be at risk for heart disease. You will find yourself still lacking energy. The key here is to be honest with yourself. Do not sugarcoat the situation.

Uncover your Motivation to Exercise

You need to uncover your motivation for exercise to stay on the right track or you will increase your chances of skipping it the very moment it starts feeling like it is a job. What inspires you to get healthier?

Does your family inspire you? Do you want to make sure that you're around for your kids as they grow up?

Are you looking to gain more energy so that you can be more productive?

There are so many factors that might motivate us that it's impossible to review them all. To change your behavior, you will need to identify patterns and then uncover why they exist. Once you start making these changes, your goals will seem much more compelling.

Stop Weighing Success on a Scale

A scale is a helpful tool for measuring your success, but you should not fall into the habit of weighing yourself every day. It is a good idea to check your weight every two weeks. Put the scale away so that you're not tempted to step on it. When you check your weight loss daily, it's much more difficult to see your progress. You will lose motivation and the slightest increase can cause you to lose motivation. It is normal for your weight to fluctuate from day to day.

Take Daily Photos

A picture is worth a thousand words, so it's really powerful to see pictures as you progress along your weight-loss journey. Build a motivational weight-loss gallery! Track your progress by creating a log that shows your weight loss over time. Consider posting these pictures on social media. When you commit to a new lifestyle publicly, you have a much higher chance of success. Being able to see the results of your diet is one of the most motivational tools you can possess.

Surround Yourself with Healthy Foods

So many have fallen off the wagon because they kept junk food around their home and eventually gave in to their temptation. Stock your kitchen with healthy foods while getting rid of all unhealthy choices. You can also decorate your kitchen with beautiful fruit bowls. There are so many steps you can take to motivate yourself into staying on top of your new lifestyle.

Use Technology to Your Advantage

There are thousands of weight loss apps available for your smartphone so you can quite literally pull motivation out of your pocket. I mean, there is an exercise app called "Zombies, Run" where you are running from zombies in a game of survival. My point is that motivation is not too difficult to find in today's world.

Face Your Fears Early

It might not be your lack of motivation, but fears that are keeping you from reaching your goals. If you find yourself struggling to stick to your plan, then you need to uncover the underlying reason. Why do you keep failing? A lot of the time, we discover hidden fears that are buried deep within us. For instance, some people worry about what others might think about their new diet. Or they perhaps they are too embarrassed to exercise in front of other people. Whatever the case, you need to face these fears early. Share your new dieting plan on Facebook. Pair with a friend for your gym visits. Just remember that you're going to receive unsolicited advice from people you barely know.

Go Online for Support

The Atkins Diet is not about promoting foods of a particular brand name or getting you to pay big money for groceries or meal plans. You can find everything you need in a handy book like this one and, for additional support, you can always go online and find chat groups or forums.

There are also many amazing and creative recipes which should ensure that you have fun while you are on this restrictive diet. You can also think about getting some of the free apps, like "MyFitnessPal", for meal tracking as they might come in handy.

LOW CARB RECIPES

21 BREAKFAST RECIPES

BREAKFAST RECIPES FOR PHASE 1

MEXICAN-STYLE EGGS ON CANADIAN BACON

Prep time: 20 min

Servings: 2

Per Serving: Carbs: 2 g, Fat: 36.5 g, Protein: 43.5 g, Calories: 516

Ingredients

- 6 ounces ground beef (80% lean / 20% fat)
- 1/2 cup green chili peppers (canned)
- 1/4 tsp garlic powder
- 1 tsp chili powder
- 1/4 tsp cumin
- 1/4 tsp leaf oregano
- 1/4 tsp salt
- 1/4 tsp black pepper
- 4 slices Canadian bacon
- 4 large eggs (whole)
- 1/2 cup, shredded cheddar cheese
- 4 sprigs cilantro

Directions

1. Spray a medium skillet with non-stick cooking spray and brown the beef over medium heat.
2. Stir in chilies, garlic powder, chili powder, cumin, oregano, salt, and pepper. Cook 5-10 minutes to blend the flavors.
3. Place the slices of Canadian bacon over the top of the beef mixture to warm. Remove pan from heat and set aside.
4. In a separate skillet, scramble eggs until set (If you prefer, you can fry or poach eggs and place on top of the beef mixture in step 5.)
5. Place 1 piece of warmed Canadian bacon on each plate, top with a quarter of the beef mixture and a quarter of the eggs. Sprinkle with cheese and chopped cilantro.

~

DEVILED EGGS

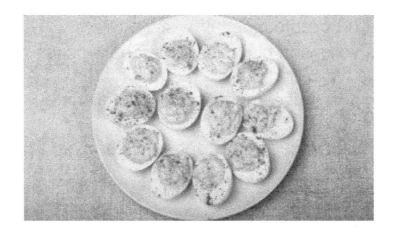

Prep time: 30 min

Servings: 1

Per Serving: Carbs: 2 g, Fat: 26 g, Protein: 25 g, Calories: 365

Ingredients:

- 4 Jumbo Eggs (Hard boiled and peeled)
- 2 tbsp. Stone Ground Mustard
- 2 tbsp. Dill Relish
- 2 tbsp. mayonnaise
- Paprika (to taste)

Directions:

1. Cut each hard-boiled egg lengthwise.
2. Remove the yolks and place inside a food processor.
3. Set aside the white portion of the egg for later.
4. Add in the mayonnaise, mustard and dill relish.
5. Blend the mixture until smooth.
6. Using a spatula, place scoops of the mixture into the white egg halves.
7. Sprinkle paprika for added flavor on top of the mixture.

TOMATO, GREEN CHILI AND CHORIZO FRITTATA

Prep time: 25 min

Servings: 6

Per Serving: Carbs: 3 g, Fat: 24 g, Protein: 22.2 g, Calories: 325

Ingredients

- 12 whole eggs
- 6 oz. beef and pork chorizo
- 8 oz. canned green chili pepper
- 2/3 cup, red tomatoes (chopped/sliced)
- 2 oz. cheddar cheese

Directions

1. In a large non-stick skillet, sauté the beef and pork chorizo at medium-high heat for about 5 minutes, breaking it down into bite-sized pieces. Remove excess fat and set aside.
2. Meanwhile, preheat the broiler.
3. Add tomatoes, lightly beaten eggs, cheese and green chilies to the chorizo in the skillet. Cook over high heat for 5 minutes and then place the skillet under the broiler for another 5 minutes or until slightly puffed. Serve immediately.

ITALIAN SQUASH PIE

Prep time: 45 min

Servings: 8

Per Serving: Carbs: 4.3 g, Fat: 14.7 g, Protein: 7 g, Calories: 176

Ingredients:

- 4 tbsp. butter
- 1 ½ lbs. yellow, summer squash (sliced thinly)
- 1 small onion (chopped finely)
- 1 clove garlic (minced)
- ½ tsp. salt
- 1.2 tsp. Italian seasoning
- ¼ cup parsley (chopped)
- 1 cup Monterey jack cheese (shredded)
- 2 eggs
- ¼ cup heavy cream
- 2 tsp. Dijon mustard

Directions:

1. Preheat the oven to 375°F .
2. In a large saucepan sauté in butter the following: squash, onion, and garlic.
3. Cook until tender and lightly browned.
4. Sprinkle in the seasoning while cooking.
5. In a greased 10-inch quiche pan, place the squash mixture.
6. Add in cheese and parsley.
7. In a small bowl, whisk the eggs and cream together.
8. Add in the mustard and blend well.
9. Pour in this mixture over the quiche pan and fold in gently.
10. Bake in the oven for about 25 minutes.
11. Once done, allow the pan to cool on a rack before cutting the pie.

WARM CHICKEN SALAD

Prep time: 40 min

Servings: 4

Per Serving: Carbs: 17 g, Fat: 30 g, Protein: 19 g, Calories: 430

Ingredients:

- 250 grams of Chicken breast (skinless and boneless)
- ½ head Lettuce
- ½ head cabbage
- 1 cucumber (sliced into cross sections)
- 1 onion (chopped)
- 5 cherry tomatoes (sliced in half)
- 1 avocado (chopped)
- ½ cup egg mayonnaise
- 2 tbsp. balsamic vinegar
- Ground coriander (for seasoning)
- Salt (for seasoning)
- Black pepper (for seasoning)
- 2 tbsp. Olive oil

Directions:

For the chicken:

1. Take the chicken breast and coat it in a mixture of salt, pepper and coriander.
2. Once coated, take a frying pan and heat the olive oil over medium heat.
3. Fry the chicken until crisp and golden brown.

For the dressing:

- Mix together egg mayonnaise and balsamic vinegar.
- Taste and adjust accordingly.

Assembly:

- Once the chicken is cooked, slice into strips.
- Place all ingredients in a mixing/salad bowl together with the chicken.
- Add the dressing on top and toss the salad lightly.
- Serve and enjoy.

MINUTE ALMOND COCONUT MUFFIN

Prep time: 5 min

Servings: 1

Per Serving: Carbs: 3.4 g, Fat: 16.8 g, Protein: 9.7 g, Calories: 208

Ingredients

- 1 large egg
- 2 tbsp. almond meal flour
- ½ tsp. cinnamon
- 1 tsp. sucralose based sugar substitute
- 1/3 tbsp. coconut flour (organic & high fiber)
- 1/8 tsp. salt
- ¼ tsp. baking powder
- 1 tsp. extra virgin olive oil

Directions

- Add all the dry ingredients in a coffee mug and stir well to
- combine. Next, add extra virgin oil and the egg to the mixture and stir until thoroughly combined.
- Microwave the mixture for a minute! Finally, use a knife to remove the muffin from the cup. Slice it and butter well to eat.

GOOD MORNING ATKINS WAFFLES

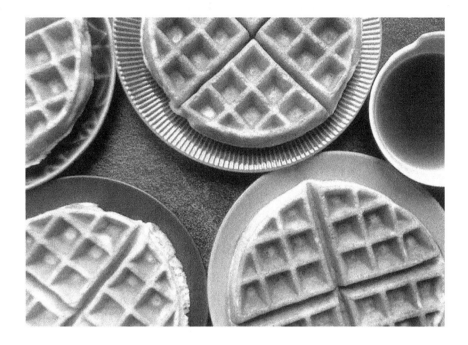

Prep time: 20 min

Servings: 5

Per Serving: Carbs: 5.7 g, Fat: 9.1 g, Protein: 14.1 g, Calories: 163

Ingredients

- 1 large egg (whole)
- 1 pack sucralose based sugar substitute
- 2 tsp. baking powder
- 1 cup cream
- ½ tsp. salt
- 3 servings soy flour, whole grain

Directions

1. In a large bowl, add 1 cup soy flour, salt sugar substitute, and baking powder. Blend the ingredients and mix well.
2. In another bowl, whisk the whole egg together with cream.

3. Add liquid ingredients to the dry ingredients and beat the batter well until there are no more lumps. Make sure you do not overbeat the mixture.
4. In order to activate the baking powder, allow the mixture to sit for at least 5 minutes.
5. In the meantime, heat the waffle iron and add the batter in the center of the iron.
6. Gently, close the top and let the waffles cook for 2 minutes or until they turn golden brown in color.
7. Enjoy!

~

BREAKFAST RECIPES FOR PHASE 2

CHEESY SAUSAGE AND EGG SCRAMBLE

Prep time: 15 min

Servings: 2

Per Serving: Carbs: 5.4 g, Fat: 19 g, Protein: 17.5 g, Calories: 267

Ingredients:

- 2 eggs
- 2 pork sausage links
- ¼ cup Cheddar cheese, shredded
- ¼ cup milk

Directions:

1. Cook sausage over medium heat or until evenly browned, in a large skillet.
2. Chop into bite-sized pieces after draining.
3. Beat milk and eggs together as the sausage is cooking.
4. Sear the eggs and add the cheese.
5. Continue cooking until eggs are set and make sure to serve warm.
6. Enjoy!

THE GREAT GAZPACHO

Prep time: 180 min

Servings: 3

Per Serving: Carbs: 13.5 g, Fat: 2.2 g, Protein: 3.5 g, Calories: 79

Ingredients:

- 1 tbsp. of fresh lime juice
- 1 garlic clove
- ¼ cup sweet onion, chopped
- 1 English Cucumber (peeled and coarsely chopped)
- 1 red bell pepper (seeded and coarsely chopped)
- 500 grams of tomatoes (cored and chopped)
- 3 tbsp. red wine vinegar
- 1 tsp. olive oil
- 2 tbsp. of fresh parsley (chopped)
- ¾ to 1 tsp kosher salt
- 2 cups tomato juice
- Red pepper flakes
- Ground black pepper

Directions:

1. In a blender, place tomatoes, cucumber, pepper, garlic clove, onion, tomato juice, olive oil, lime juice, and herbs. Process the mixture until smooth.
2. Then, add red pepper flakes, kosher salt, and vinegar and process until you reach your desired taste.
3. Chill in the fridge overnight. You can also just refrigerate it for around 2 to 4 hours, if desired.
4. Drizzle olive oil on top and garnish with green onion, chopped peppers, and black pepper.
5. Serve and enjoy!

BREAKFAST STUFFED PEPPER, MEXICAN STYLE

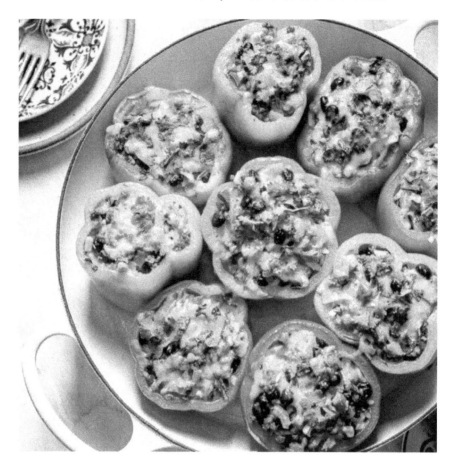

Prep time: 45 min

Servings: 1

Per Serving: Carbs: 3.7 g, Fat: 24.5 g, Protein: 15 g, Calories: 300

Ingredients

- 1 oz. pork and beef chorizo
- 1 ounce 80% lean ground beef
- 2 tablespoons chopped onion
- ¼ oz. cheddar cheese, grated
- 1 large egg, beaten
- 1 medium sweet red peppers, cut in half lengthwise, seeds and white ribs removed

Directions

- Preheat oven to 400°F and line a baking sheet with foil.
- In a pan over medium heat, cook chorizo and ground beef, crumbling meat while it cooks. Drain off excess fat.
- Place cooked meat mixture in mixing bowl and combine with the onion, cheese and egg.
- Fill pepper half with the meat mixture and place on the prepared baking sheet. Bake for 25-30 minutes and serve hot.

BREAKFAST YOGURT WITH ALMOND SURPRISE

Prep time: 5 min

Servings: 1

Per Serving: Carbs: 10.7 g, Fat: 3 g, Protein: 21 g, Calories: 145

Ingredients:

- 1 cup Greek or plain yogurt (kept cold for at least 30 minutes)
- 1 tsp. ground cinnamon
- 3 tbsp. almonds (roasted, unsalted and slivered)

Directions:

1. In a small cereal bowl, place the yogurt, cinnamon and almonds.
2. Mix well and serve.

BLACKBERRY SMOOTHIE

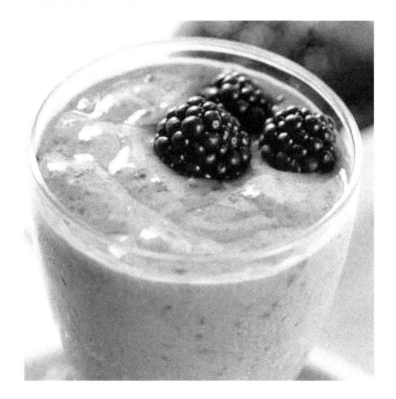

Prep time: 5 min

Servings: 1

Per Serving: Carbs: 6 g, Fat: 6.9 g, Protein: 25 g, Calories: 210

Ingredients

- ¼ cup frozen blackberries
- 1 cup unsweetened coconut, almond, or soy milk
- 1 oz. vanilla whey protein
- 1 tablespoon ground golden flaxseed meal
- ¼ tsp cinnamon
- pinch ground allspice
- ½ teaspoon vanilla extract

Directions

1. Combine the frozen blackberries, milk, protein powder, flax meal, vanilla, and spices in a blender.
2. Blend until smooth.

LOW-CARB CHEESE BREAD SNACK

Prep time: 35 min

Servings: 5

Per Serving: Carbs: 7.2 g, Fat: 12 g, Protein: 11 g, Calories: 177

Ingredients:

- 1 cup of soy flour
- 1 tsp. of baking powder
- ½ tsp. of salt
- ½ cup of shredded cheddar
- 1 egg (slightly beaten)
- ¼ cup of cream

Directions:

1. Preheat the oven at 350°F.
2. Take a baking sheet and place wax paper over it.
3. In a mixing bowl, sift all of the dry ingredients together to remove any lumps.
4. Mix in the cheese.
5. Fold in the egg and cream as you continue to mix the ingredients.
6. Continue to beat the mixture until smooth.
7. Take the mixture out of the bowl and roll into an 8x8" square.
8. Cut the square into 1" sized cubes.
9. Place each individual cube onto the baking sheet.
10. Sprinkle with a dash of salt.
11. Place in the oven and bake for about 10 minutes or until golden brown.

SMOKED SAUSAGE WITH SPECIAL DIP

Prep time: 15 min

Servings: 4

Per Serving: Carbs: 18 g, Fat: 37 g, Protein: 33 g, Calories: 535

Ingredients:

- 16 oz. smoked sausage (halved lengthwise and then sliced into bite size pieces)
- 2 tbsp. Dijon mustard
- 3 tbsp. horseradish
- 2 cups shredded cheddar cheese
- ½ cup mayonnaise
- 1 cup green onions (chopped)

Directions:

1. In a large, non-stick skillet, fry the sausages for about 3 to 5 minutes or until they change color.
2. Once cooked, remove excess oil using a paper towel.
3. Mix the rest of the ingredients in a bowl and heat in the microwave for about 60 seconds.
4. Stir the mixture until smooth. If lumps are still present, heat again if necessary. Enjoy!

~

BREAKFAST RECIPES FOR PHASE 3

PEAR AND PECAN SALAD

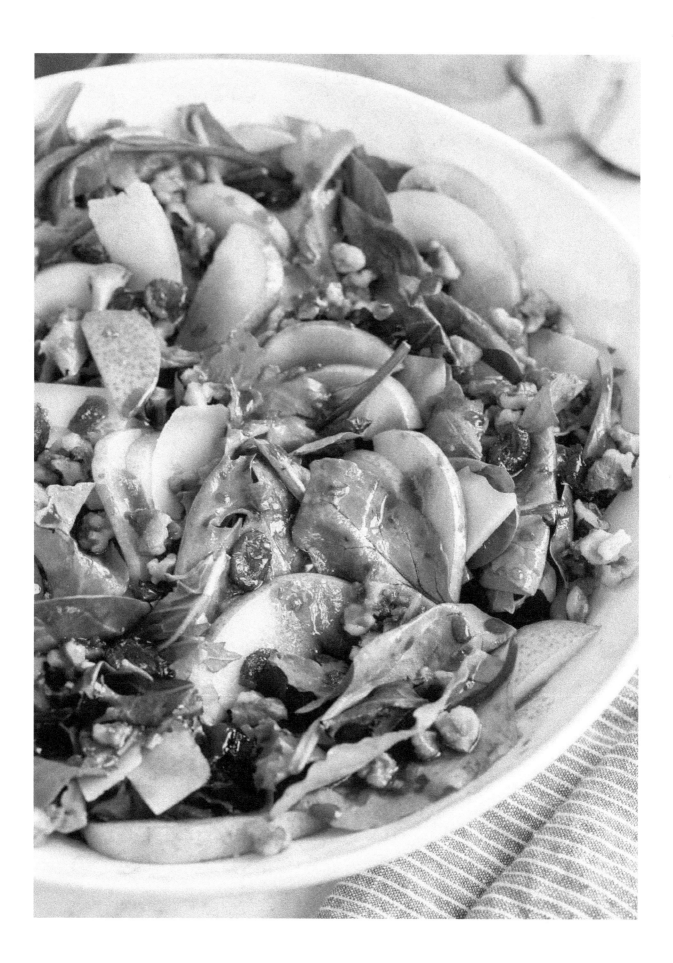

Prep time: 30 min

Servings: 6

Per Serving: Carbs: 8 g, Fat: 18.6 g, Protein: 5.1 g, Calories: 224

Ingredients:

- ½ cup of Gouda cheese
- ½ cup of pecans (halved)
- 1 tbsp. of unsalted butter
- 3 tbsp. of walnut oil
- 1 medium sized pear (sliced into wedges)
- 1/8 tsp. curry powder
- ¾ tsp. of salt
- ¼ tsp. freshly ground black pepper
- ¾ cup of wine vinegar
- 2 tsps. of sucralose sweetener
- 10 cups of salad leaves (lightly packed)
- 1/8 tsp. of red pepper
- ¾ cup of white wine vinegar

Directions:

Spiced pecans:

1. In a medium sized non-stick skillet, melt the butter over medium heat.
2. Add in the pecans, 1 tsp. of the sucralose, salt and cayenne pepper.
3. Stir the mixture using a wooden spoon for about 4-5 minutes, or until the pecans are toasted evenly.
4. Make sure that the nuts are coated well with the spices.
5. Set aside in a small bowl to cool.

Salad dressing:

1. In a medium sized mixing bowl, add the remaining tsp. of sucralose together with salt, vinegar, pepper and curry powder.
2. Mix well until the powder has been dissolved.
3. With a wire whisk, beat the mixture slowly as you add in the walnut oil.
4. Continue whisking until dressing is smooth.

In another salad bowl, place the salad leaves, Gouda cheese and pear wedges.

1. Pour in the salad dressing and lightly toss.
2. Serve with spiced pecans on the side or placed in an entirely separate bowl.

GREEN TEA INFUSED CANTALOUPE SOUP

Prep time: 20 min

Servings: 4

Per Serving: Carbs: 11 g, Fat: 1.3 g, Protein: 0.6 g, Calories: 61

Ingredients:

- 1 and ½ cups of cantaloupe (Cubed/ Diced)
- ½ cup of brewed green tea (cooled to room temperature)
- 1 tsp. of fresh mint sprigs

Directions:

1. Place in a blender the diced cantaloupe.
2. Blend well until puréed. As the blender is running, gradually add in ½ cup of green tea.
3. Continue blending until smooth and free of lumps.
4. Take a spatula and spoon out the mixture into 4 separate soup bowls.
5. Garnish with mint sprigs on the side.

QUICK AND EASY SEARED SCALLOPS

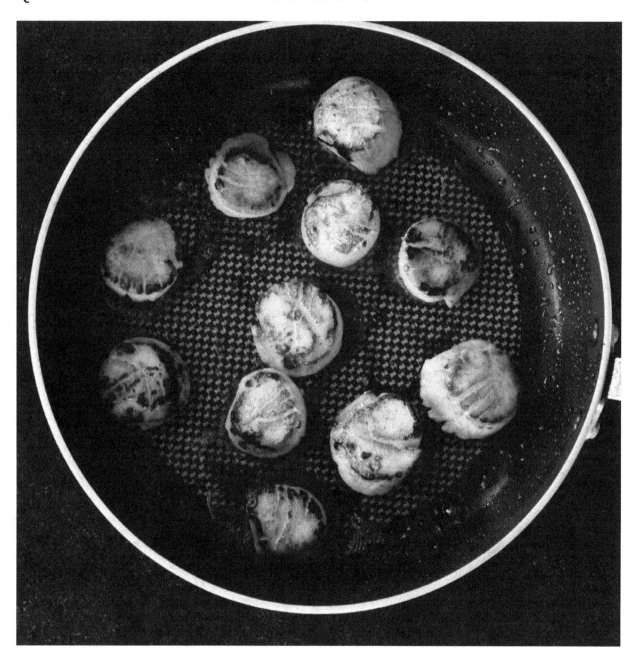

Prep time: 15 min

Servings: 3

Per Serving: Carbs: 10.5 g, Fat: 5.3 g, Protein: 34 g, Calories: 225

Ingredients:

- 1 Tbsp. of butter
- 500 grams of sea scallops
- Salt and pepper, to taste

Directions:

1. Roll both sides of the scallops onto salt and pepper and dry on paper towels.
2. Then, heat pan for around 2 to 3 minutes or until hot.
3. Add butter then add the scallops and make sure that they do not touch each other.
4. If you can't cook them all at once, just place some of them on a large piece of foil and cook them in batches. 2 batches of these shall be okay.
5. Then, cook each side of the scallop for around 1 to 2 minutes or until center is translucent. Make sure that both ends are golden. Use tongs to turn.
6. Serve immediately and enjoy!

~

BRAISED SHORT RIBS WITH HORSERADISH SAUCE

Prep time: 180 min

Servings: 4

Per Serving: Carbs: 7 g, Fat: 24 g, Protein: 30.5 g, Calories: 326

Ingredients

- 3 pounds short ribs
- ½ teaspoon sea salt
- ¼ teaspoon black pepper
- 1 ½ teaspoons canola oil
- 1 cup chopped fennel
- 1 medium carrot, finely diced
- 2 large garlic cloves, minced
- ½ cup plus 2 tablespoons dry red wine
- 14 oz. can beef broth
- ¼ teaspoon ground allspice
- 2 tablespoons whole wheat flour

For horseradish cream:

- ½ cup sour cream
- 1 tablespoon prepared white horseradish, well drained
- 1 tablespoon thinly sliced scallions

Directions:

1. Preheat oven to 350°F. Sprinkle short ribs with salt and pepper. On the stove, set burner to medium high heat and set Dutch oven on burner. Place half of ribs in Dutch oven and brown well, about 3 to 4 minutes per side. Transfer to a plate and repeat with remaining ribs, removing them when they're browned.
2. Reduce heat to medium. Add oil, fennel, and carrot to Dutch oven and

cook for about 3 minutes, or until vegetables are light golden. Add garlic and cook for 1 minute. Add ½ cup wine and simmer for 1 minute. Add ribs to vegetable/wine mixture and stir in broth and allspice. Bring to a boil.

3. Cover and transfer to preheated oven for 2 ¼ to 2 ½ hours, until meat is so tender it falls off the bone.

4. While ribs are braising, prepare horseradish cream. Mix sour cream, horseradish, and scallions. Stir until combined. Store in refrigerator until serving time.

5. 5.When ribs are done, transfer to a bowl. Skim as much fat as possible from the surface of the liquid. (Can be made a day ahead and refrigerated so that the fat hardens and is easily removed.)

6. Stir remaining 2 tablespoons of wine into flour and whisk into cooking liquid. Bring to a boil and simmer 1 to 2 minutes until thickened, stirring frequently. Return ribs to liquid and cook until heated through. Serve with horseradish cream.

COWBOY BREAKFAST SKILLET

Prep time: 30 min

Servings: 5

Per Serving: Carbs: 12 g, Fat: 17 g, Protein: 22 g, Calories: 355

Ingredients

- 1 lb. breakfast sausage
- 2 medium sweet potatoes, diced
- eggs
- 1 avocado, peeled and cubed
- handful cilantro, chopped
- hot sauce
- ½ cup grated cheese (optional)
- salt and pepper to taste

Directions

1. Preheat oven to 400ºF.
2. In a cast iron or other oven-safe skillet, crumble and brown the sausage over medium heat. Use a slotted spoon to remove the sausage and drain on paper towels. Leave as much of the sausage drippings as possible in the skillet.
3. Add the sweet potatoes to the skillet and toss in the sausage grease until cooked through and crispy.
4. Return the sausage to the pan, and with a large spoon, make a depression in the mixture, a "nest" for each egg. Crack your eggs into the nests.
5. Place the skillet into the preheated oven and bake just long enough for the eggs to set (about 5 minutes).
6. Now, turn the oven to broil the top of the eggs for a few minutes, but don't let the yolk cook all the way through–unless you prefer a well-cooked yolk. Remove the pan from the oven and top with avocado,

cilantro, and hot sauce.

7. Use a large spoon to scoop out each egg, along with its nest.

CHEESE BAKED ATKINS EGGS

Prep time: 15 min

Servings: 1

Per Serving: Carbs: 2 g, Fat: 27.6 g, Protein: 17 g, Calories: 327

Ingredients

- 2 whole eggs
- 1 tsp. butter stick (unsalted)
- 2 tbsp. heavy cream
- 2 tbsp. grated parmesan cheese

Directions

1. Coat the inside of an oven safe dish with melted butter.
2. In a medium bowl, add heavy cream and eggs and whip together lightly.
3. Add salt, freshly ground pepper and parmesan cheese as per your taste.
4. Bake in the oven at 375°F for about 10 minutes or until set.
5. Enjoy!

BROCCOLI AND ARUGULA SALAD

Prep time: 5 min

Servings: 4

Per Serving: Carbs: 5 g, Fat: 10 g, Protein: 1 g, Calories: 120

Ingredients:

- 3 T extra virgin olive oil
- 2 T sherry vinegar or apple cider vinegar
- ½ t black pepper
- ⅜ t kosher salt
- 3 c baby arugula
- 1 ½ c broccoli slaw mix
- 1 c shredded carrot

Directions

1. Combine first 4 ingredients and mix well with a whisk.
2. Mix arugula, broccoli slaw mix, and carrot.
3. Pour dressing over salad and toss lightly until coated.

21 LUNCH RECIPES

LUNCH RECIPES FOR PHASE 1

SHRIMP FRIED "RICE"

Prep time: 15 min

Servings: 4

Per Serving: Carbs: 6 g, Fat: 17 g, Protein: 20 g, Calories: 269

Ingredients:

- 3 tablespoons toasted sesame oil, divided
- 10 oz. medium shrimp, peeled and deveined
- 5 large eggs, lightly beaten
- 1 cup sliced green onions, divided
- 16 oz. fresh or frozen riced
- cauliflower ½ t freshly ground
- black pepper ¼ t kosher salt

Directions

1. Heat 1 ½ teaspoons sesame oil in a large nonstick skillet over medium high. Add shrimp and cook 3 minutes. Remove shrimp from pan.
2. Return pan to medium high. Add 1 ½ teaspoons oil. Add eggs, cook 2 minutes or until almost set, stirring once. Fold cooked eggs in half; remove from pan. Cool and cut into ½ inch pieces.
3. Heat remaining 2 tablespoons of oil in pan over medium-high. Add ¾ cup of green onion, cauliflower. Cook 5 minutes without stirring or until browned. Stir in shrimp, eggs, salt, and pepper. Top with remaining ¼ cup green onions.

POACHED CHICKEN

Prep time: 20 min

Servings: 3

Per Serving: Carbs: 3 g, Fat: 14 g, Protein: 31 g, Calories: 260

Ingredients:

- 1 lb. chicken breast (should be boneless and skinless)
- 3 strips of lemon zest (Remove with a knife or vegetable peeler)
- 1 piece fresh or dried bay leaf

Directions:

1. In a shallow pot with tight fitting lid, place the chicken inside.
2. Fill the pot with enough water to cover the chicken completely.
3. Add in the lemon zest and bay leaf. Cook slowly over medium heat.
4. Allow the pot to simmer before reducing the heat to low.
5. Make sure that the water produces small bubbles.
6. Partially cover the pot and allow to cook for 10 minutes or until the chicken is tender.
7. To check if your chicken is cooked thoroughly, take a fork and pierce the middle portion. The chicken should release clear juices.
8. Using a sieve, take the chicken out of the pot and place on a plate with a paper towel.
9. Drain the chicken of any excess juices before transferring to a serving plate.

GOOD NOON TUNA KEBABS

Prep time: 30 min

Servings: 4

Per Serving: Carbs: 3.9 g, Fat: 3 g, Protein: 28.8 g, Calories: 178

Ingredients

- 16 oz. raw tuna, boneless
- 2,5 tbsp. tamari soy sauce (gluten-free)
- ½ tbsp. ginger
- 1 fl. oz. rice wine
- 1,5 tsp. garlic
- ½ tbsp. sesame oil, toasted
- 1 tsp. sucralose based sugar substitute
- 1,5 spring onions or scallions
- ½ lb. eggplant
- Handful of red sweet pepper
- 4 metal skewers

Directions

1. Pre-heat the grill to high heat.
2. In a large mixing bowl, combine sesame oil, ginger, soy sauce, rice wine, sugar substitute, garlic and ginger.
3. After some time, add scallions, tuna and red pepper; toss well to coat together. Allow it to marinate for about 10-15 minutes in the refrigerator. Remove and set aside.
4. Put the eggplant in marinade and allow it to sit for 5 minutes to make sure it is well-coated. Remove eggplant and set it aside for further use. Discard the marinade.
5. Thread metal skewers, alternating 2 pieces of scallions and red pepper each, 3 pieces of tuna, and 3 pieces of eggplant on each. Remember: Skewer the eggplant through both skin sides of the rounds.

6. Grill for about 4-5 minutes each side making sure tuna isn't at the center of the grill.
7. Remove and serve immediately.

SALMON CROQUETTES

Prep time: 20 min

Servings: 2

Per Serving: Carbs: 2.8 g, Fat: 21 g, Protein: 50 g, Calories: 415

Ingredients:

- 1 15oz. can of salmon (drained)
- 2 tbsp. soy flour
- 1 egg
- ¼ cup green onion (minced)
- Salt and pepper (for seasoning)
- Olive oil

Directions:

1. In a medium bowl, place the salmon.
2. Remove any bones and skin.
3. Mash the salmon using a fork before adding in the following: flour, egg, and onions.
4. Add salt and pepper to taste.
5. Form small patties, using the mixture.
6. Each patty should be around 2 inches in diameter. In a medium sized skillet, heat 2 tbsp. of olive oil and fry the patties over medium heat until patties are golden brown or crisp on the outside.
7. Be careful not to burn them.
8. Once cooked evenly, place on a paper towel to drain excess oil.
9. Serve with hot sauce or sour cream.

~

BRUSSELS SPROUTS WITH BACON AND PARMESAN

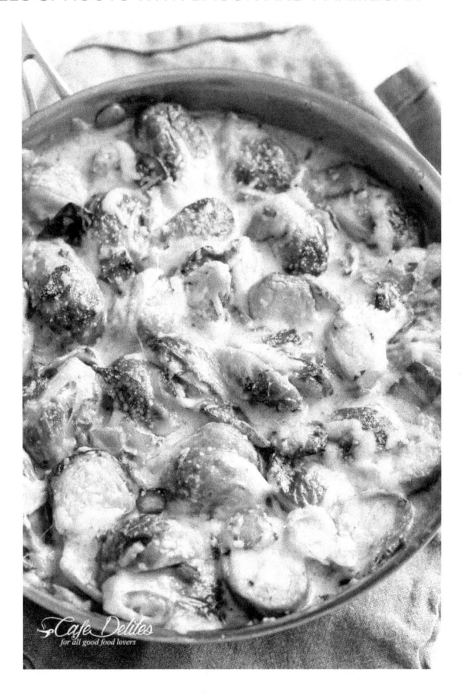

Prep time: 30 min

Servings: 6

Per Serving: Carbs: 4.3 g, Fat: 8.1 g, Protein: 7 g, Calories: 128

Ingredients

- 6 oz. raw bacon
- 2 lbs. brussels sprouts
- 1 tsp. sea salt
- ½ cup freshly grated parmesan cheese
- 1 tsp. ground black pepper
- ½ cup heavy whip cream

Directions

1. Rinse and pat dry the brussels sprouts with a paper towel. Now, cut them in half.
2. In a medium sized skillet, cook bacon over medium-high heat until it turns brown. Transfer it on a paper towel when done and set aside to let cool.
3. In a different skillet, add salt, pepper, brussels sprouts, Add brussels sprouts and sauté over medium-high heat, stirring occasionally for 15 minutes or until lightly golden.
4. Add parmesan cheese and heavy whip cream to the skillet, and stir to heat for another 1 minute.
5. Transfer to a serving bowl and top with bacon. Serve immediately.

COUNTRY STYLE GARDEN PASTA SALAD

Prep time: 40 min

Servings: 3

Per Serving: Carbs: 15 g, Fat: 9.6 g, Protein: 22 g, Calories: 240

Ingredients:

- ¼ cup penne pasta
- 250 grams of chicken breast (boneless, skinless, cooked and shredded)
- ¼ medium sized red onion (thinly sliced)
- ¼ cup of blue cheese (crumbled)
- ½ cup of fresh blueberries
- 2 tbsps. of olive oil
- 2 tbsps. of freshly squeezed lime juice
- 1 pinch of sucralose
- 1 tbsp. lime zest
- 1 tbsp. of fresh thyme (finely chopped)

Directions:

1. Prepare the pasta according to the package instructions and set aside for later.
2. Place the shredded, cooked chicken in a shallow bowl and combine with onions, blue cheese and blueberries.
3. Mix thoroughly all the ingredients (by hand or using a spatula). Set aside.

For the dressing:

1. In a small mixing bowl, pour in the olive oil and lime juice.
2. Gradually whisk in the sucralose, thyme, and lime zest.
3. Season it with salt and pepper.

4. Mix thoroughly.
5. Take the dressing and pour over the cooked pasta.
6. Lightly toss to coat the pasta evenly.
7. Transfer the pasta with dressing in a serving dish. Add the chicken mixture on top.

COCO LOCO SHRIMP

Prep time: 15 min

Servings: 2

Per Serving: Carbs: 3 g, Fat: 13 g, Protein: 55.7 g, Calories: 368

Ingredients:

- 1 lb. large, raw shrimp, deveined and peeled
- ¼ tsp black pepper
- ¼ tsp cayenne pepper
- 1/3 cup of coconut flour
- vegetable oil
- 2 eggs
- ½ cup coconut, shredded and unsweetened
- 2 tbsp. water
- Sucralose (optional)
- 1 tsp salt

Directions:

1. Combine flour with salt and red peppers.
2. Then, in a small dish, whisk eggs with 2 tablespoons of water.
3. In a separate dish, place the shredded coconut then heat some oil in a skillet.
4. Heat skillet to 350°F and wait for some bubbles to form.
5. Roll shrimp in coconut flour by the tail and then shake off excess flour.
6. Dip it into the egg and shake off any excess liquid away before rolling it in the coconut flour once more.
7. Fry each side of the shrimp for 2 minutes and make sure to do it in small batches so as not to crowd the pan. Use some tongs to flip the shrimp.
8. Remove the shrimp from the pan after frying and let it cool in a wire

rack. Serve with your choice of sweet or spicy sauce and enjoy!

LUNCH RECIPES FOR PHASE 2

STIR-FRIED STEAK WITH ASPARAGUS

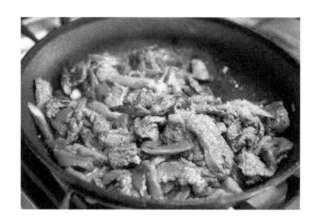

Prep time: 15 min

Servings: 2

Per Serving: Carbs: 11 g, Fat: 33 g, Protein: 39 g, Calories: 15

Ingredients:

- 12 oz. sirloin steak, boneless, and cut into ¼ inch strips
- 5 tsp canola oil, divided
- 1 tsp cornstarch
- 2 tsp garlic, minced
- 2 tsp fresh ginger, peeled and grated
- 1 ½ Tbsp. soy sauce (low sodium variety)
- 1 ½ tbsp. oyster sauce
- ¼ cup chicken stock, unsalted
- 1 red bell pepper, medium, cut into strips
- 1 ¼ cup of medium asparagus, cut into 2 inch pieces
- 3 green onions, chopped
- ½ tsp red pepper, crushed

Directions:

1. Combine chicken stock, oyster sauce, fresh ginger, garlic, and soy sauce in a bowl. Stir with a whisk.
2. Heat skillet over high heat and add a teaspoon of oil into the skillet.
3. Add beef and stir-fry until browned.
4. Move beef onto another plate and discard the liquid.
5. Add 2 more tablespoons of oil into the pan.
6. Add bell pepper and asparagus and stir-fry for 2 more minutes then turn the heat down to medium-high.
7. Pour stock mixture into the skillet and cook until sauce is thick or for around 3 minutes.
8. Add juices back to the pan and continue cooking for another minute.
9. Serve and enjoy!

VEGGIE TUNA SALAD

Prep time: 5 min

Servings: 4

Per Serving: Carbs: 17 g, Fat: 22 g, Protein: 22.2 g, Calories: 370

Ingredients:

- 6 plum tomatoes (chopped)
- 8 ribs leafy celery (chopped)
- 1 medium onion (chopped)
- 1 can of chickpeas (drained)
- ½ cup black olives (pitted and chopped coarsely)
- ½ cup of fresh parsley leaves (chopped)
- 2 lemons
- 2 cans tuna, drained and flaked
- 1/3 cup of olive oil

Directions:

1. Combine chickpeas, tomatoes, celery, olives, parsley, and onion in a bowl, then add tuna flakes and mix until well-combined.
2. Add lemon juice and olive oil to the salad and mix well.
3. Season the salad with salt and pepper before serving. Enjoy!

FANTASTIC POTATO GNOCCHI

Prep time: 100 min

Servings: 2

Per Serving: Carbs: 30 g, Fat: 21 g, Protein: 12 g, Calories: 370

Ingredients:

- 80 grams almond flour
- 330 grams yellow potatoes
- Nutmeg (ground)
- Salt (to taste)

Directions:

1. Peel the potatoes and chop into cubes.
2. Place them in a pressure cooker and steam for 10 minutes
3. Once the potatoes have cooled, mash them with a fork or potato masher.
4. Make sure to remove lumps. Season with nutmeg and salt.
5. Sprinkle flour onto your working surface and place the mashed potatoes there.
6. Add the rest of the flour and make dough.
7. Cut the dough into at least 6 sections and roll each to create a sausage-like shape.
8. Cut the "sausage" every 2 centimeters and add more flour, if necessary.
9. You may choose to add ridges to the gnocchi with the use of a fork or grater.
10. You may also make them hollow by pressing them. Put the gnocchi in the fridge for at least an hour.
11. After an hour, boil gnocchi in salted water until they float.
12. After float, drain gnocchi and season with the dressing of your choice.

ATKINS CHICKEN VEGGIE BOWL

Prep time: 20 min

Servings: 3

Per Serving: Carbs: 2.5 g, Fat: 7.4 g, Protein: 10.6 g, Calories: 103

Ingredients

- 3 cups chicken broth
- 1,5 cups spring onions or scallions (chopped)
- 1 cup mushroom stems and pieces
- 1 minced garlic clove
- 1,5 tsp. ginger
- 2 tbsp. tamari soybean sauce
- Handful serrano pepper
- ½ cup tomatoes (chopped/ sliced)
- 3 oz. silken tofu
- 1 large carrot
- ¼ oz. coriander (cilantro)
- ½ cup cabbage (shredded)

Directions

1. In a large skillet, add chicken broth and tamari sauce; bring to a boil.
2. Slightly reduce the heat; add mushrooms, cabbage, minced garlic, ginger, and chili. Simmer the mixture for the 5 minutes or until the cabbage is tender and the mushrooms have softened.
3. Add spring onions, tomatoes, carrot and tofu and heat for another 1 minute.
4. Stir in cilantro and serve warm.

~

MOVER MUFFINS

Prep time: 20 min

Servings: 8

Per Serving: Carbs: 19 g, Fat: 7 g, Protein: 6 g, Calories: 166

Ingredients:

- 1 scoop of protein powder
- ¼ cup of oat bran
- 1 cup of bran
- ½ cup of cream
- 1 large egg
- ½ cup of sucralose
- 1 tsp. vanilla extract

Directions:

1. Preheat the oven to 350°F before you begin.
2. In a mixing bowl, combine the oat bran, bran, cream, and sucralose.
3. Beat in the egg with the mixture.
4. As you mix, gradually add in the protein powder, little by little.
5. Take a muffin tray and line with cooking spray.
6. Bake in the oven for about 15 minutes

COCONUT PIE

Prep time: 65 min

Servings: 8

Per Serving: Carbs: 20 g, Fat: 14 g, Protein: 3.7 g, Calories: 224

Ingredients:

- 4 large eggs
- 1 cup of water
- 4 tbsp. of butter
- ½ cup of almond flour
- 1 cup of heavy cream
- 3 tsp. of vanilla extract
- ¾ cups of sucralose
- 1 cup of fresh coconut (shredded)

Directions:

1. Preheat the oven to 350°F.
2. Take a 9" pie dish and grease using cooking spray.
3. In a large mixing bowl, combine together butter and eggs.
4. Beat together until creamy.
5. Add in cream, vanilla extract and water.
6. Gradually fold the almond flour and sucralose into the mixture.
7. Mix well until smooth.
8. Add in the shredded coconut and mix for another 2 minutes.
9. Pour the contents of the bowl into the pie dish and bake in the oven for about 1 hour or until the mixture sets.
10. Place on a wire rack to cool before serving.

~

SWEET AND SPICY CHICKEN

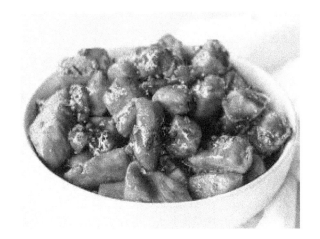

Prep time: 510 min

Servings: 4

Per Serving: Carbs: 9 g, Fat: 4.7 g, Protein: 43 g, Calories: 256

Ingredients:

- 1 kg chicken breasts
- ¼ tsp. cayenne pepper
- 2 tsp. garlic, chopped
- ¼ cup fresh orange juice
- 1 tsp. orange peel, grated
- 1 tsp. granular sugar substitute
- 1 tbsp. chili powder

Directions:

1. Mix orange juice, chili powder, garlic, cayenne pepper, orange rind, and sugar substitute in a re-sealable plastic bag.
2. Add chicken breasts and toss until well coated. Keep in the fridge for around 6 to 8 hours or overnight.
3. Season chicken with salt and pepper and heat the broiler.
4. Place chicken in the broiler and broil for at least 12 to 15 minutes.

5. Turn chicken after 6 minutes and cook each side until browned or cooked through.
6. Enjoy!

LUNCH RECIPES FOR PHASE 3

SPANISH VEGETABLES WITH CAULIFLOWER MASH

Prep time: 60 min

Servings: 2

Per Serving: Carbs: 15 g, Fat: 0.6 g, Protein: 4.3 g, Calories: 94

Ingredients:

- 1 head of cauliflower (grated)
- 1 bell pepper (roughly diced)
- ½ cup of onions (roughly diced)
- Olive oil
- 1 cup of fresh whole tomatoes (canned can also be used)
- 1 tbsp. of balsamic vinegar
- 1 tsp. Worcestershire sauce
- 1 tsp. of sucralose
- Salt and pepper (to taste)
- 2 green scallions (finely chopped)

Directions:

1. In a medium sized saucepan over medium heat, mix the following ingredients together: tomatoes, vinegar, Worcestershire sauce, sucralose, salt and pepper.
2. Using a wooden spoon, break the tomatoes into smaller chunks.
3. Cover the pan and allow the mixture to simmer for 30 minutes. Do not let the mixture dry out.
4. While the mixture simmers, take a large skillet and over medium to high heat, cook the bell peppers and onions.
5. Allow them to get slightly charred before taking out of the heat. Place about a teaspoon of olive oil to the skillet then add in the grated cauliflower.
6. Stir the mixture thoroughly and continue to cook for about 3 minutes or until the cauliflower becomes soft with the consistency of mash.
7. If it takes too long, you may opt to cover the skillet for a few minutes to hasten the process.
8. Place in a bowl or serving dish and then top of with the tomato sauce and chopped scallions.

MEXICAN SURPRISE

Prep time: 55 min

Servings: 4

Per Serving: Carbs: 29 g, Fat: 11 g, Protein: 25 g, Calories: 328

Ingredients:

- 1/3 cup of salsa
- 1 cup cheddar cheese (shredded)
- ½ cup reduced fat sour cream
- 1 cup of skim milk
- 1 whole egg
- 3 egg whites
- 6 oz. ground turkey sausage
- 5 slices brown bread (cubed)

Directions:

1. Spray a pie plate with cooking spray.
2. Place the bread cubes evenly in the pie plate and set them aside.
3. Cook sausage in medium-high heat in a skillet until browned. Break up the pieces as needed.
4. Place the sausage on top of the bread cubes. Beat the egg whites together with milk, whole egg, and sour cream in a bowl.
5. Add cheese and mix until well combined.
6. Pour this cheese and egg mixture over the sausage. Refrigerate for at least 2 hours or overnight.
7. After taking it out of the fridge, bake for approximately 35 minutes in an oven at 325°F and let the mixture stand for around 10 minutes after removing from the oven. After 10 minutes, cut the bread.
8. Serve each slice with some salsa on top. Enjoy!

MACARONI SALAD WITH A TWIST

Prep time: 55 min

Servings: 4

Per Serving: Carbs: 22 g, Fat: 25 g, Protein: 2,8 g, Calories: 330

Ingredients:

- 1 ½ cups of penne pasta
- 2 cups of cauliflower (chopped coarsely)
- ½ cup of mayonnaise
- 2 tbsp. of Dijon mustard
- 2 tsps. of Sucralose
- 1/3 cup of celery (finely chopped)
- ¼ cup of dill pickles (finely chopped)
- ¼ cups of fresh olives

Directions:

1. Prepare the pasta according to the package instructions and set aside.
2. Take the pasta out of the water and place in a separate dish.
3. Keep the pasta water.
4. Add the cauliflower to the pasta water and boil until cauliflower becomes tender.
5. Set aside to cool.

For the dressing:

1. Take a large mixing bowl and combine mayonnaise, sucralose and Dijon mustard.
2. Whisk together until blended before adding in chopped celery, pickles and olives.
3. Add pasta and cauliflower. Using a spatula, fold in the pasta gently until it is coated evenly.

4. Add salt and freshly ground black pepper to taste.

TURNIPS AND CAVIAR AFTERNOON SNACK

Prep time: 20 min

Servings: 1

Per Serving: Carbs: 16 g, Fat: 16 g, Protein: 6,1 g, Calories: 230

Ingredients:

- 4 small turnips (peeled and sliced)
- Olive oil
- Caviar

Directions:

1. Preheat the oven to 400°F.
2. Place some olive oil in a small bowl and dip the turnips in the oil.
3. Place the oil-coated turnips on a baking sheet coated with wax paper.
4. Season turnips with salt and pepper.
5. Bake turnips for about 15 minutes or until golden brown.
6. Make sure to flip the turnips so they bake evenly on each side.
7. Once baked, serve with a little sour cream and a small amount of caviar on top.

PEACHY PROSCIUTTO BITES

Prep time: 25 min

Servings: 1

Per Serving: Carbs: 4.5 g, Fat: 21.3 g, Protein: 14 g, Calories: 269

Ingredients

- 6 thin slices prosciutto
- ½ medium sized peaches
- 1 tsp. ground cinnamon
- 2 oz. cream cheese
- ¼ cup almonds (whole)
- 6 basil leaves

Directions

1. Preheat oven to 350°F. Toast nuts for 10 minutes before coarsely chopping them into smaller pieces. Likewise, slice the peach into 6 smaller slices and set aside.
2. In a medium-sized mixing bowl, combine 1 tsp. cinnamon with the softened cream cheese and a pinch of stevia (optional). Now, add the nuts and blend well to combine.
3. Place 1 tbsp. of cheese mixture on top of each peach wedge and dress with a basil leaf at the top. Lay a single slice of prosciutto flat, placing the peach wedge at one end of the prosciutto and rolling-it-up.
4. Repeat the same step with the remaining ingredients. Remember: 1 serving = 3 peach wedges.

BAKED CATFISH WITH BROCCOLI AND HERB-BUTTER BLEND

Prep time: 15 min

Servings: 1

Per Serving: Carbs: 3.8 g, Fat: 25.8 g, Protein: 29 g, Calories: 370

Ingredients:

- 1 cup chopped broccoli
- 1 serving Herb-Butter Blend
- 6 oz. channel catfish (farmed)

Directions

Cooking fish in an aluminum-foil packet makes for easy cleanup and works especially well for single portions. Add a vegetable and you have a complete quick meal. Use butter or 1 tablespoon of the Atkins recipe: Herb-Butter Blend.

1. Preheat oven to 350°F.
2. Place the catfish on a 12-inch square piece of foil. Sprinkle fish with salt and freshly ground pepper to taste. Arrange broccoli florets around fish.
3. Fold up the sides of the foil and crimp tightly to form a sealed packet.
4. Bake for 10-15 minutes until fish is flaky and broccoli is tender.
5. Transfer to a dish, open foil and top with a tablespoon of Herb-Butter Blend.

ACORN SQUASH WITH SPICED APPLESAUCE AND MAPLE DRIZZLE

Prep time: 30 min

Servings: 8

Per Serving: Carbs: 22 g, Fat: 5 g, Protein: 2 g, Calories: 141

Ingredients

- 1 4 inch acorn squash
- 5 tablespoons unsalted butter
- ½ teaspoon salt
- ½ teaspoon black pepper
- ¾ cup unsweetened applesauce
- ⅛ teaspoon cinnamon
- 1 tablespoon sugar-free maple flavored syrup

Directions

1. Preheat oven to 350°F. Cut squash in half, remove seeds, and then cut into six wedges.
2. Line a sheet pan with aluminum foil. Melt 1 tablespoon butter and brush on squash; sprinkle with salt and pepper, place on pan, and bake in preheated oven until squash is fork tender (about 20 minutes).
3. In a small saucepan, heat the applesauce for about three minutes. Stir in 2 teaspoons butter and cinnamon and cook 30 seconds more.
4. Serve squash with a dollop of apple sauce mixture and a drizzle of about 1/2 teaspoon syrup.

21 DINNER RECIPES

DINNER RECIPES FOR PHASE 1

FAUX MASHED "POTATOES"

Prep time: 30 min

Servings: 1

Per Serving: Carbs: 4 g, Fat: 5.5 g, Protein: 2.4 g, Calories: 80

Ingredients

- 1 cup cauliflower florets
- 1 tablespoon butter
- 2 tablespoons heavy cream
- sea salt
- ground pepper

Directions

1. Steam cauliflower florets until tender.
2. Puree with butter and cream.
3. Season to taste with salt and pepper.

CREAMY SOUP WITH MINI TURKEY MEATBALLS

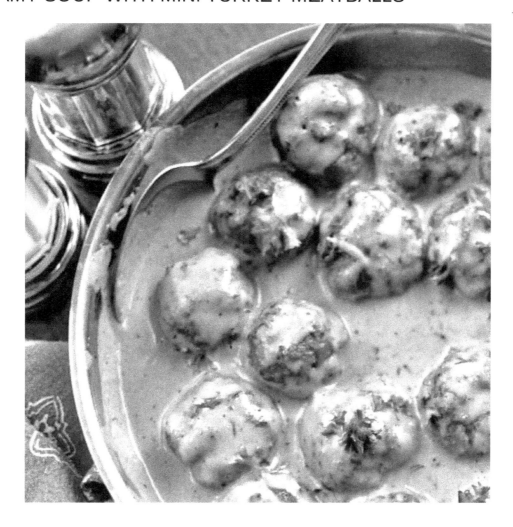

Prep time: 30 min

Servings: 2

Per Serving: Carbs: 3 g, Fat: 27.8 g, Protein: 27.2 g, Calories: 382

Ingredients

- 1 tbsp. unsalted butter
- 1 minced clove garlic
- 1 ¼ oz. chopped broccoli
- about 4 medium white mushrooms,
- chopped 8 oz. lean ground turkey 1
- extra large egg
- 1 tablespoon chicken bouillon
- ¼ cup heavy cream
- spices to taste for meatballs (suggestion: chili powder, oregano, ground ginger, ground curry, turmeric, basil)
- enough water to cook mini-meatballs in.

Directions

1. Bring water to a boil.
2. In a small bowl, combine ground turkey, egg, and spices. Working with tablespoon-sized scoops, form the mixture into small balls and set aside.
3. Melt butter in medium saucepan and add garlic. Stir over medium heat for about 30 seconds and then add the mushrooms. Allow them to cook down and add the chopped broccoli.
4. Add about 5 cups boiling water to the sautéed veggies. Bring to boil again and add the bouillon. Water can be increased or decreased according to taste.
5. Drop the meatballs into the boiling soup mixture. Let cook for about 10 minutes and then add the heavy cream. Taste and adjust seasoning if necessary.

SPINACH CUPS

Prep time: 30 min

Servings: 8

Per Serving: Carbs: 3.6 g, Fat: 0.2 g, Protein: 1.6 g, Calories: 22

Ingredients:

- 2 egg whites (slightly beaten)
- ¼ cup pimientos (chopped)
- 2 whole green onions (thinly sliced)
- 1 tbsp. of fresh parmesan cheese (grated)
- 1 1/3 cups spinach (chopped)
- Salt and pepper (to taste)

Directions

1. Preheat the oven to 350°F.
2. Take one ¾" muffin tin and line with cooking spray.
3. In a mixing bowl, combine the egg whites, pimientos, green onions and parmesan cheese.
4. Add salt and pepper to adjust the taste.
5. Mix well using a spatula. Add in the spinach.
6. Using a mixer or blender, blend all the ingredients together until smooth.
7. Take the mixture and fill in the muffin tins until 2/3 of the way.
8. Grate some parmesan cheese on top before baking in the oven for 10 minutes.

CHEESY KALE AND TOMATO CHIPS

Prep time: 12.5 hours

Servings: 4

Per Serving: Carbs: 20,2 g, Fat: 17 g, Protein: 11 g, Calories: 257

Ingredients:

- 30 grams organic tomatoes, sun-dried, and soaked for around an hour in water
- 1 bunch kale, leaves ripped and stems removed
- 2 large garlic cloves
- 1 cup raw cashews,
- 2 to 4 tbsp. fresh basil
- ¾ cup + 2 tbsp. tomato soaking water
- ¾ tbsp. sea salt
- 2 tbsp. nutritional yeast
- 2 tbsp. fresh lemon juice

Directions:

1. Soak cashews together with the tomatoes for around an hour in water to soften.
2. Set aside the soaking water after taking the cashews and tomatoes out.
3. Pulse garlic in a food processor until thoroughly minced.
4. Add the rest of the ingredients with the exception of salt and process until smooth. Add salt, to taste.
5. After washing kale leaves, tear them into pieces and discard the stems.
6. You can place the leaves in a salad spinner to dry.
7. Pour the cheesy sauce that you have made over the kale and stir until well coated.
8. Place kale in a dehydrator and process at 110 F for around 12 hours.
9. Once the chips are crispy, it means that they're ready to serve.

BUFFALO HOT WING CAULIFLOWER

Prep time: 55 min

Servings: 4

Per Serving: Carbs: 7 g, Fat: 16 g, Protein: 6.5 g, Calories: 204

Ingredients

- 1 cauliflower head (large)
- 2 tbsp. extra virgin olive oil
- 4 tbsp. buffalo hot wing sauce
- 2 tbsp. butter stick (unsalted)
- 2 tsp. sriracha chili sauce
- 1 ¼ oz. Roquefort or blue cheese

Directions

1. Preheat oven to 375°F.
2. Chop the large cauliflower head into smaller florets and drizzle with 1 tbsp. olive oil. Let it roast on a baking sheet for half an hour or until tender.
3. In the meantime, put sriracha and buffalo hot wing sauce in a small sauce pan at medium heat and bring to boil for 10 minutes. Add butter and stir until melted. Allow the mixture to cool at room temperature.
4. Pour the remaining 1 tbsp. olive oil into a large saucepan and bring to a boil. Add the cauliflower florets prepared in step 2 and sauté until they are heated thoroughly. Add the sauce mixture while continuing to cook for another 1 minute.
5. Top with Roquefort or blue cheese and serve immediately.

APPLE STUFFED CHICKEN BREAST

Prep time: 35 min

Servings: 4

Per Serving: Carbs: 2.5 g, Fat: 13 g, Protein: 73 g, Calories: 420

Ingredients:

- 800 grams of chicken breast (boneless, skinless and cooked)
- ¼ cup almonds (sliced or slivered)
- 2 tbsp. of olive oil
- ½ tsp. of garlic (minced)
- 3 tbsps. of fresh parsley (finely chopped)
- ¼ tsp. of salt
- ¼ tsp. of freshly ground black pepper
- 1/3 cup of apples (peeled, cored and finely chopped)
- 1 cup of mozzarella cheese

Directions:

1. Preheat the oven to 350°F.
2. Place almonds on a baking sheet or skillet.
3. Add a drizzle of olive oil and then toast in the oven for 3 minutes.
4. Set aside to cool.

For the stuffing:

1. Mix in a small bowl the following: cheese, apples, garlic, almonds, parsley, salt and pepper.
2. Mix the ingredients using a spatula or by hand.
3. Take the chicken breasts and create pockets for the stuffing by slicing lengthwise cuts into each piece.
4. Rub salt and pepper on each piece of chicken to season.
5. Take a spoon and add stuffing to each piece of chicken. Be sure to

add just enough stuffing that you will still be able to close it.
6. Secure the pocket opening by inserting a toothpick on the open end.

Over medium-high heat, cook the chicken breast in a medium sized skillet for about 5 minutes or until clear juices come out of the chicken. Place in a serving dish and serve.

ALMOND BALLS

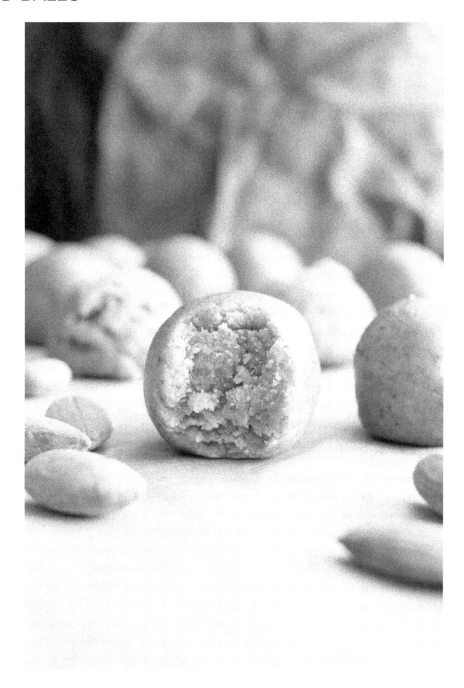

Prep time: 20 min

Servings: 24

Per Serving: Carbs: 1.7 g, Fat: 4.3 g, Protein: 2.1 g, Calories: 55

Ingredients

- 1 whole egg
- 1 egg yolk
- ½ cup blanched almonds
- ¾ cup soy flour, whole grain
- 3 tsp. baking powder
- ¾ cup sucralose based sugar substitute
- 2 tsp. vanilla extract
- ¼ cup butter stick (unsalted)

Directions

1. Preheat oven to 375°F.
2. In a blender, finely grind soy flour with the almonds, sugar substitute and baking powder.
3. In a separate bowl, using an electric mixer, beat egg yolk, whole egg, butter and vanilla on medium until well incorporated. Spoon in the soy mixture with a rubber spatula.
4. Use your hands to form 24 small balls out of the dough; and arrange them on a baking sheet.
5. Bake in a preheated oven for 10 minutes or until set. Let it cool on baking sheets before serving or refrigerate overnight.

CREAMED CABBAGE WITH CHILIES AND GINGER

Prep time: 40 min

Servings: 5

Per Serving: Carbs: 15.6 g, Fat: 5 g, Protein: 4 g, Calories: 110

Ingredients:

- 3 pcs crystallized ginger (about the size of a quarter)
- 3 small red chilies (dried)
- 1 large heads of savoy cabbage (thinly sliced; crosswise)
- ¾ cups whipping cream
- 1,5 tbsp. butter
- ½ tbsp. white wine vinegar
- 1 tbsp. grated orange peel (optional)
- ½ cup of fresh basil leaves (thinly sliced)

Directions:

1. In a medium sized bowl, combine the ginger and chilies.
2. Place enough boiling water to cover the mixture.
3. Leave for 15 minutes.
4. Drain the water, but set aside ¼ cup of the liquid.
5. Take the contents of the bowl and pour into a blender.
6. Puree until smooth and free of lumps.

In a separate pot,

1. Boil cabbage in salted water for about 2 minutes.
2. Drain the cabbage and let it cool down by running it through cold water.

3. Mix the following in a saucepan: whipping cream, butter and vinegar.
4. Bring to a boil.
5. Allow the mixture to thicken for about 3-5 minutes.
6. Fold in the chili puree.
7. Add the cabbage and orange peel.
8. Stir under low heat.
9. Add in the basil.
10. Add salt and pepper to taste.
11. Adjust accordingly.

GRANDMA'S RUSTIC COLE SLAW WITH WALNUTS

Prep time: 35 min

Servings: 8

Per Serving: Carbs: 12.7 g, Fat: 6.8 g, Protein: 3.5 g, Calories: 124

Ingredients:

- 2/3 cup of vinegar
- 2 large eggs (lightly beaten)
- A pinch of salt (to taste)
- ½ cup of whipping cream
- ¼ cup of Sucralose
- 1 head of cabbage (shredded)
- 1 and ½ tbsp. of butter (cut into small chunks)
- ½ cup of walnuts (chopped)

Directions:

1. In a small, heavy-bottomed saucepan, combine the vinegar, whipping cream, eggs, sucralose and salt.
2. Stir constantly using a whisk over low heat for about 10 minutes or until the mixture becomes thickened.
3. Once the consistency is right, remove the pan from heat. Add in the butter and continue stirring until completely melted.
4. In a mixing bowl, place the cabbage and walnuts.
5. Pour in the mixture to coat the cabbage.
6. Lightly toss. Cool to room temperature before covering and placing in the fridge to chill.

THE BEST HOMEMADE TOTS

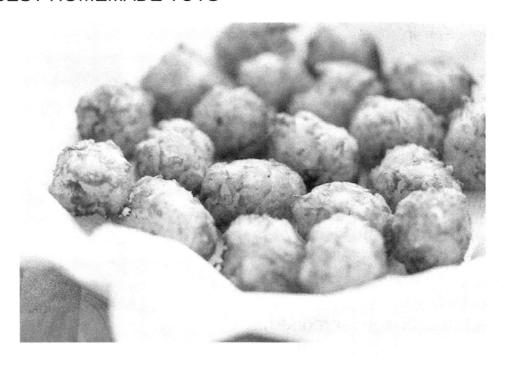

Prep time: 25 min

Servings: 4

Per Serving: Carbs: 46 g, Fat: 2 g, Protein: 7 g, Calories: 247

Ingredients:

- 3 tbsp. onion (finely chopped)
- 6 small potatoes (peeled and cubed)
- 1 large egg
- ¼ cup flour
- Kosher salt
- Vegetable oil
- Pepper
- 1 tbsp. rosemary

Directions:

1. In a large pot, cook potatoes in salted water until tender.

2. After cooking, drain the potatoes and place them in a ricer, with the help of a bowl.
3. Grate the onion over the bowl and add it to the potatoes.
4. Add egg, flour, and rosemary.
5. Season with pepper and salt and mix until well combined.
6. Roll the potatoes on a floured surface and cut into tots.
7. Then, pour oil on a countertop fryer and heat to 350 F.
8. In small batches, fry the tots for around 4 minutes or until golden and crispy and drain on paper towels.
9. Season tots with salt and serve.

BLACK BEANS AND QUINOA

Prep time: 45 min

Servings: 4

Per Serving: Carbs: 33 g, Fat: 4 g, Protein: 10 g, Calories: 232

Ingredients:

- 1 onion, chopped
- 1 tsp vegetable oil
- 1 tsp ground cumin
- 1 ½ cups vegetable broth
- ¾ cup quinoa
- 3 cloves garlic (chopped)
- ½ cup fresh cilantro (chopped)
- 2 cans black beans, rinsed and drained
- 1 cup of corn kernels
- ¼ tsp cayenne pepper
- Ground black pepper and salt, to taste

Directions:

1. In a saucepan, heat oil over medium heat and add onions.
2. Cook for around 10 minutes or until onions are lightly brown.
3. Stir occasionally.
4. Then, add quinoa and vegetable broth into the onions and season with cayenne pepper, cumin, black pepper, and salt.
5. Boil mixture and reduce heat after covering.
6. Simmer for around 20 minutes or until tender.
7. Make sure that the broth has been absorbed.
8. Add frozen corn and simmer for around 5 minutes or until heated through.
9. Add cilantro and black beans and mix until well combined.
10. Serve and enjoy!

SUPER STACKED EGGPLANTS

Prep time: 70 min

Servings: 4

Per Serving: Carbs: 12 g, Fat: 32 g, Protein: 13 g, Calories: 387

Ingredients:

- 3 tbsp. red wine vinegar
- 6 ½ tbsp. olive oil
- 1 tbsp. dried oregano
- 1 large clove of garlic (pressed)
- 1 tsp. salt
- ¼ cup pumpkin seeds (toasted)
- ¼ cup parmesan cheese (grated)
- 1 cup of basil leaves
- 1 eggplant (cut into 1 to 1 ½ inch thick pieces)
- 1/8 tsp ground black pepper
- 4 oz. fresh mozzarella (sliced thinly)
- 1 medium tomato (sliced thinly)
- 1 tsp balsamic vinegar

Directions:

1. In a large bowl, combine red wine vinegar, olive oil, oregano, garlic, salt and pepper altogether.
2. Then, add eggplant and toss until well combined.
3. Let the mixture stand for at least an hour, occasionally turning the eggplant.
4. Pulse parmesan, basil, pine nuts, and olive oil in a food processor until pasty. Transfer to a bowl and cover with plastic wrap.
5. In a pie plate, combine balsamic vinegar, ¼ oil, and ½ teaspoon of salt together with sliced tomato and a pinch of black pepper.
6. Mix until tomatoes are well coated.

7. Arrange the pieces by placing eggplant slices on a platter and spreading ½ teaspoon of pesto on top of each.
8. Top with a slice of tomato and a slice of mozzarella.
9. Add pesto, eggplant, cheese and tomato. Drizzle eggplant stacks with any remaining juice from cooking.
10. Serve and enjoy!

ROASTED VEGETABLES IN HERBS

Prep time: 40 min

Servings: 1

Per Serving: Carbs: 42 g, Fat: 0.6 g, Protein: 4.8 g, Calories: 224

Ingredients:

- 1 small red onion (sliced)
- 1 medium parsnip (peeled and cut into 1 inch pieces)
- 2 carrots (peeled and cut into 1 inch pieces)
- 2 medium sweet potatoes (cut into 1 inch cubes)
- ½ tsp ground black pepper
- ½ tsp salt
- 2 tsp basil
- 2 tsp thyme
- 2 tsp oregano
- 3 cloves garlic (minced)

Directions:

1. Pre-heat the oven to 425°F.
2. Place carrots, potatoes, onion, and parsnip in a baking dish.
3. Mix herbs, garlic, oil, pepper, and salt in a medium bowl and pour the mixture over the vegetables. Mix until well coated.
4. Bake for approximately 30 minutes, covered. Bake until you reach your desired tenderness.
5. Stir vegetables and bake for 10 minutes more.
6. Serve and enjoy!

ASPARAGUS WRAPPED IN CHILI SPICED BACON

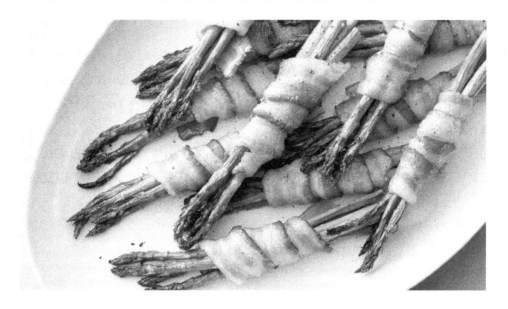

Prep time: 20 min

Servings: 4

Per Serving: Carbs: 1.8 g, Fat: 2.2 g, Protein: 4 g, Calories: 46

Ingredients:

- 1 tsp chili powder
- 1/2 teaspoon Sucralose based
- sweetener 4 slice bacon
- 24 spear asparagus

Directions:

1. Soak 16 wooden toothpicks in warm water for 20 minutes.
2. Preheat grill. Place a sheet of wax paper on a sheet pan and set aside. Combine the chili powder and sugar substitute in a small bowl.
3. Cut bacon strips in 1/2. Lay them on the sheet pan and dust with the chili powder mixture.
4. Wrap three asparagus spears together with one slice of bacon (with the dusted side facing towards the asparagus); secure each end with a toothpick. You should have 8 packets.
5. Grill uncovered over medium-low heat for 12 minutes turning halfway through or until bacon is crisp.
6. Discard toothpicks and serve immediately. Each serving is 2 wraps.

DINNER RECIPES FOR PHASE 3

QUICK BAKED TOFU WITH MOROCCAN RUB

Prep time: 35 min

Servings: 1

Per Serving: Carbs: 5.9 g, Fat: 9.8 g, Protein: 12.5 g, Calories: 153

Ingredients

- 6 oz. tofu (firm and silken)
- 1 tsp. extra virgin olive oil
- 1 tbsp. Moroccan rub

Directions

1. Rinse the tofu and pat dry it with a paper towel. Chop it into strips of ¼" inch.
2. Rub the tofu strips with 1 tbsp. Moroccan rub combined with 1 tsp. olive oil and let it marinate for 30 minutes.
3. Preheat oven the oven to 375°F.
4. Grease a flat pan with some olive oil and bake tofu on it for 15 minutes.
5. Flip it over and bake for another 15 minutes or until it turns golden brown in color and appears crisp.

CREAMY GREEN BEANS

Prep time: 15 min

Servings: 1

Per Serving: Carbs: 23 g, Fat: 20 g, Protein: 8.5 g, Calories: 290

Ingredients:

- 4 tbsp. double cream
- 5 tbsp. sour cream
- 300 grams green beans
- Zest of ½ lemon
- 2 tbsp. Dijon mustard
- 1 tbsp. capers, chopped

Directions:

1. Cook the beans in boiling water for 5 minutes.
2. Combine capers, sour cream, double cream, mustard and lemon zest altogether.
3. After cooking the beans, season them with salt and pepper add then add to cream mixture.

RED GRAPEFRUIT SALAD

Prep time: 25 min

Servings: 4

Per Serving: Carbs: 16 g, Fat: 10 g, Protein: 2 g, Calories: 160

Ingredients:

- 2 pcs. of white grapefruit (sectioned)
- 2 pcs. of red or pink grapefruit (sectioned)
- 1 tsp. tarragon leaf
- ¼ tsp. of yellow mustard seeds
- 3 tbsps. olive oil
- 5 cups of mixed fresh salad leaves
- ½ of a small red onion (chopped)

Directions:

1. Section each grapefruit by removing the outer covering and membranes.
2. Squeeze out all remaining juice and set aside in a small bowl for later use.

For the dressing:

1. In a small mixing bowl, take 1 tbsp. of the grapefruit juice and mix together with mustard seeds.
2. Whisk together with olive oil until evenly blended.
3. Add in tarragon, salt, and freshly ground pepper for seasoning.
4. Taste and adjust accordingly.

In another salad bowl,

1. Place the salad leaves, red onion and grapefruit sections together.
2. Pour in dressing and lightly toss.

BRISKET WITH MUSHROOMS

Prep time: 125 min

Servings: 10

Per Serving: Carbs: 2.4 g, Fat: 36 g, Protein: 34.4 g, Calories: 485

Ingredients

- 15 individual pieces of porcini mushrooms (dried)
- 1 tbsp. extra virgin olive oil
- 4 lbs. whole beef brisket (diced to 1/8" fat)
- 2 medium onions
- 1 ½ tsp. garlic
- 1 14 oz. can beef broth
- 1 tsp. bay leaf (crumbled)
- ¼ tsp. black pepper
- ½ tsp. salt

Directions

1. In a small bowl, add ¾ cup of water and mushrooms. Microwave on high for about 2-3 minutes or until water boils. Remove the mushrooms, set them aside and let them cool to room temperature. Mince garlic, dice the onions, and set them aside.
2. In a large Dutch oven, heat the extra virgin olive oil over medium heat. Add brisket and let it brown on one side. Flip it over, add chopped onions and continue to brown. Once onions are brown, add minced garlic. Cook for another 1 minute.
3. Rinse the mushrooms, chop them and place into the Dutch oven.
4. Add bay leaf, beef broth, salt, and pepper. Cover the oven, slightly reduce the heat to low and cook for about 2 hours or until brisket turns tender. Now, transfer the brisket to a cutting board.
5. Meanwhile, increase the heat to high and let the juices thicken. Take out the bay leaf. Cut the brisket into thin slices and enjoy it with the

mushroom gravy.

BLACKENED ATKINS SALMON

Prep time: 11 min

Servings: 4

Per Serving: Carbs: 0.2 g, Fat: 24 g, Protein: 37 g, Calories: 372

Ingredients

- 3 tsp. dried thyme
- 3 tsp. oregano leaves
- 1 tbsp. old bay seasoning
- 1 tsp. freshly ground black pepper
- 1 tsp. salt
- 6 tbsp. vegetable oil
- 24 oz. salmon, raw and boneless

Directions

1. In a small mixing bowl, combine oregano leaves, dried thyme, salt, pepper and the Old Bay seasoning.
2. Coat each piece of salmon with 2 tbsp. vegetable oil; and rub the mixture prepared in step 1 into flesh of the fish on both sides.
3. Ensuring good ventilation with an exhaust fan, heat remaining vegetable oil in a large skillet over medium to high heat. Add the spice-rubbed salmon and sear for 3 minutes on both sides or until coating turns black in color.
4. Serve right away with avocado salsa. (Refer to the snack recipe 1)

BROCCOLI FLORETS WITH LEMON BUTTER SAUCE

Prep time: 11 min

Servings: 4

Per Serving: Carbs: 7.3 g, Fat: 12 g, Protein: 3.7 g, Calories: 144

Ingredients

- 1 lb. broccoli florets
- 2 tbsp. shallots, chopped
- 1 fl. oz. wine of choice
- 1 tbsp. freshly zest lemon juice
- 4 tbsp. butter stick, unsalted
- 1/8 tsp. white pepper
- 1/8 tsp. salt

Directions

1. In a large pot, add water, salt and broccoli florets. Cook for about 5-7 minutes or until tender. Drain the water; keep the florets warm within the pot as you prepare the sauce.
2. In a small saucepan, place shallots, 1 tbsp. fresh lemon juice, and 2 tbsp. wine and heat over medium-high heat. Reduce heat to very low; mixing in some small pieces of butter and whisk until it has mostly melted.
3. Slowly and gradually, stir in the remaining butter, mixing continuously until a smooth sauce is formed. Season with remaining lemon juice, 1/8 tsp. white pepper, and 1/8 tsp. salt. Make sure the sauce doesn't boil.
4. Pour the sauce over your broccoli florets and enjoy.

ATKINS BBQ CHICKEN SUPREME PIZZA

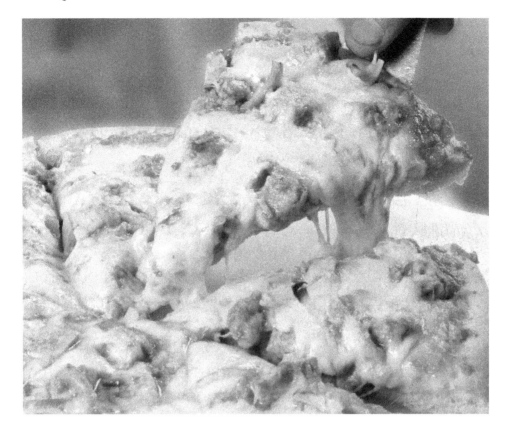

Prep time: 50 min

Servings: 8

Per Serving: Carbs: 6.3 g, Fat: 9.5 g, Protein: 8 g, Calories: 126

Ingredients

- 1 ½ tsp. baking powder
- 1 tsp. salt
- 1 packet sucralose based sugar substitute
- 1 cup tap water
- 1 red onion, small
- 1 cup chicken breasts, cooked and
- diced ½ medium sweet peppers (green)
- 1 cup mozzarella cheese, shredded
- 3 tbsp. virgin olive oil

- 6 serving's whole grain soy flour
- 2 servings BBQ sauce

Directions

1. Pre-heat the oven to 425°F.
2. In a large mixing bowl, blend together baking powder, whole grain soy flour, sugar substitute and salt.
3. Mix in oil and water and combine into the dough using a wooden spatula or spoon.
4. Transfer the dough on to a clean surface that is lightly coated with extra-virgin olive oil.
5. Spray the rolling pin with oil spray and roll out the dough until it fits the pizza pan. You can also use your hands to bring the dough into shape.
6. Transfer it to a pre-heated oven, bake for 10 minutes and remove.
7. Dress the BBQ sauce evenly over the pizza. Top with chicken pieces, sprinkle with mozzarella, onions and bell pepper slices. Season with salt and pepper to taste.
8. Return to the oven and bake for 15 minutes. Cut into 8 slices and enjoy.

7 SNACK RECIPES

ATKINS AVOCADO SALSA

Prep time: 10 min

Servings: 4

Per Serving: Carbs: 2.6 g, Fat: 6.7 g, Protein: 1.3 g, Calories: 86

Ingredients

- 1 large red tomato
- 1/8 cups coriander (cilantro)
- 1 medium red onion
- ½ jalapeño peppers
- 1 California avocado
- 2 tbsp. freshly zest lime juice
- ¼ tsp. salt
- ¼ tsp. black pepper

Instructions

1. Chop the whole tomato and coriander, set aside. Dice the jalapeno and the onion.
2. Gently remove the skin of the avocado, slice it and place in the serving bowl. Add lime juice, diced onion and jalapeño to the avocado and gently mix. Note: Do not mash!
3. Add the chopped cilantro and tomato; season with salt and pepper to taste.
4. Cover the salsa and refrigerate until you're ready to serve.

BUFFALO CHICKEN EGG SALAD

Prep time: 20 min

Servings: 8

Per Serving: Carbs: 1.1 g, Fat: 12.3 g, Protein: 11 g, Calories: 154

Ingredients

- 6 boiled eggs
- 6 oz. cooked chicken thighs (boneless)
- 3 tbsp. mayonnaise
- 1 ½ tbsp. hot buffalo wing sauce
- ¼ cup Roquefort/blue cheese (crumbled)
- 8 stalk, medium celery

Instructions

1. Hard boil the eggs: Place your eggs in a pot with water and bring to a boil over medium-high heat. Remove from heat and set aside for 10 minutes. Drain; let the eggs cool in ice water and then peel. Reserve in a medium bowl.
2. Cook chicken thighs in a large skillet over medium heat until the meat no longer remains pink in the center and the juices run clear. Transfer to the bowl with the eggs.
3. Add cheese, buffalo wing sauce and mayonnaise. Mix to combine the flavors. Sprinkle salt and pepper to taste.
4. Serve with the celery stalks.

FRENCH STYLE-QUESADILLAS

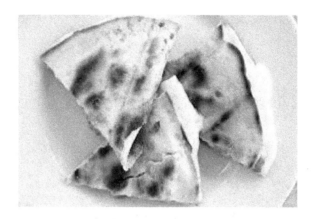

Prep time: 15 min

Servings: 4

Per Serving: Carbs: 8.7 g, Fat: 17.5 g, Protein: 18 g, Calories: 269

Ingredients

- 3 oz. cooked ham (boneless)
- 1 medium pear
- 4 oz. soft brie cheese
- 4 low carb tortillas
- ¼ cup almonds (sliced)

Instructions

1. Preheat oven to 350°F.
2. On a sheet-pan, lay the low-carb tortillas flat. Layer the ham, pear, almonds and brie cheese onto half of each tortilla.
3. Gently, fold the tortilla and bake in the preheated oven for 5 minutes.
4. Cut them in half and serve immediately.

LEMON ZEST TUNA SALAD

Prep time: 5 min

Servings: 1

Per Serving: Carbs: 4.8 g, Fat: 45 g, Protein: 45 g, Calories: 611

Ingredients

- 6 oz. canned tuna in water
- 1 ½ tbsp. fresh lemon juice
- 3 tbsp. mayonnaise
- 2 cups rocket arugula
- ½ cup cucumber, sliced
- 1 tbsp. extra virgin olive oil

Instructions

1. In a medium sized mixing bowl, combine tuna, 1 tbsp. lemon juice, and mayonnaise. Season with sea salt and freshly ground pepper as per your taste.
2. Serve over the rocket arugula and sliced cucumber sprinkled with olive oil and remaining ½ tbsp. lemon juice.

LOW CARB GRILLED CHEESE WITH TOMATO

Prep time: 10 min

Servings: 1

Per Serving: Carbs: 3.3 g, Fat: 37 g, Protein: 25 g, Calories: 450

Ingredients

- ¼ cup cheddar cheese, shredded
- 2 medium tomatoes, sliced
- 1 tsp. butter stick, unsalted
- 1 loaf low carb bread

Instructions

1. Preheat a non-stick pan over medium to high heat; add butter and let it melt.
2. Slice the low carb bread loaf into two thinner slices and add them to the pan. Let one side brown first and then flip over to brown the other side. Meanwhile, when one side browns, add cheese to the top of the opposite side (at the top) of bread slice.
3. Now, place two slices of tomato atop the bread slice with melted cheese. Season with sea salt and freshly ground black pepper to taste. Finally, place the other piece of bread on top.
4. Enjoy!

CHORIZO WITH LEMON-MAYO DIP

Prep time: 25 min

Servings: 4

Per Serving: Carbs: 2.8 g, Fat: 78 g, Protein: 22 g, Calories: 805

Ingredients

- 6 link (4" long) pork and beef chorizo
- 1 tsp. extra virgin olive oil
- 1 cup mayonnaise
- 1 fl. oz. lemon juice
- 3 tsp lemon zest
- 1/2 clove garlic
- 2 stalk, medium (7-1/2" - 8" long) celery

Instructions

1. Slice chorizo into 1/2-inch rounds. Heat oil in a large skillet over medium heat. Cook chorizo 5 to 7 minutes, turning once, until browned on both sides. Remove from pan and drain on paper towels.
2. Place mayonnaise, lemon juice, zest and minced garlic in a small bowl. Stir well to combine. Cut the celery into sticks and serve with the chorizo and dipping sauce. Chorizo may be served warm or cold.

BLACK OLIVES WITH CHEDDAR

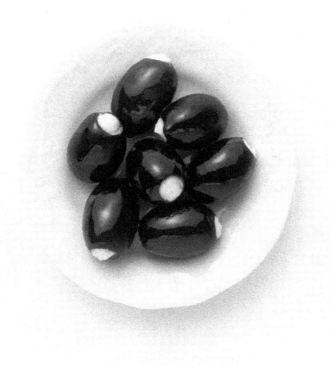

Prep time: 5 min

Servings: 1

Per Serving: Carbs: 3.6 g, Fat: 19 g, Protein: 8 g, Calories: 223

Ingredients

- 7 Greek olive black olives
- 1 slice (1 oz.) cheddar cheese

Instructions

1. Dice the cheese and place into hole of the olive.
2. Pop into your mouth and enjoy!

5 DESSERT RECIPES

ATKINS MOCHA GRANITA

Prep time: 25 min

Servings: 6

Per Serving: Carbs: 3.8 g, Fat: 0.7 g, Protein: 1.3 g, Calories: 22

Ingredients

- 1 cup of tap-water
- 1 cup of coffee
- 10 packets of sucralose based sugar substitute
- 1/3 cup unsweetened cocoa powder
- 4 tbsp. chocolate syrup (sugar-free)

Instructions

1. In a heavy saucepan, add coffee, water, and all the individual sachets of the sugar substitute and mix over medium heat. Blend in the chocolate syrup and the cocoa powder. Gently, simmer the mixture.
2. Simmer the mixture while stirring constantly for about 5 minutes. Remove from the heat and pour mixture through a fine strainer into a large measuring cup. Refrigerate for 1-2 hours or until cold.
3. Transfer the mixture into ice cube trays, filling them only half way. Freeze until firm.
4. When you are ready to serve, process the chocolate cubes in a food processor and sprinkle over the granita cubes.

PEACH BUTTERMILK SHERBET

Prep time: 40 min

Servings: 8

Per Serving: Carbs: 6 g, Fat: 12 g, Protein: 2.22 g, Calories: 166

Ingredients

- 3 medium peaches (coarsely diced)
- 1/3 cup xylitol
- 10 individual sachets of stevia
- ¼ cup freshly squeezed lemon juice
- ½ tsp. salt
- 1 cup heavy whipped cream
- 1 cup buttermilk

Instructions

1. In a large saucepan, combine peaches and stevia; cook over medium-high heat for 10-15 minutes or until tender. Allow to cool for 10 minutes.
2. In a blender, process the cooking juices and the peaches with salt and lemon juice (as per your taste). Add heavy whipped cream and buttermilk. Mix well to combine and refrigerate overnight.
3. Transfer the mixture to an ice cream maker and follow the manufacturer's directions. Once done, serve the sherbet immediately or pack into a freezer-safe container freeze it.

DOUBLE CHOCOLATE ATKINS COOKIES

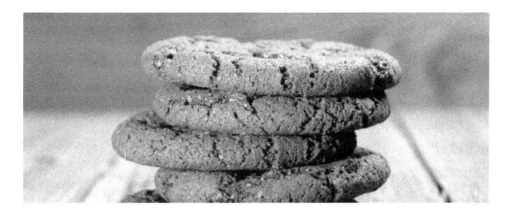

Prep time: 30 min

Servings: 18

Per Serving: Carbs: 1.3 g, Fat: 8.7 g, Protein: 2.7 g, Calories: 107

Ingredients

- ¼ cup butter stick (unsalted)
- 1 tsp. vanilla extract
- 1/3 cups powdered xylitol
- 1 large whole egg
- 1 ½ cups almond flour (blanched)
- ¼ tsp. baking soda
- 2 tbsp. unsweetened cocoa powder
- 3 packets of Indulge chocolate candies
- 1/3 tsp. salt

Instructions

1. Preheat an oven to 350°F. Use parchment paper or a silpat mat on the cookie sheet.
2. In a small bowl, beat the unsalted butter stick using the powdered xylitol for about 3 minutes or until light and fluffy. Add the whole egg and vanilla and whisk until well combined.
3. In a medium mixing bowl, add all the remaining dry ingredients except chocolate candies and stir well to combine. Add dry ingredients to the wet ingredients and blend until mixed smoothly. Add the chocolate candies and stir to combine.
4. Use your hands to roll dough to form 18 individual 1-inch balls and arrange 1-inch apart on the prepared cookie sheet. Put the balls to the pre-heated oven and bake for about 10 minutes. Remove from oven and set aside for 5 minutes before moving to the cooling rack. Cookies can either be served immediately or stored in an airtight container for up to 2 days.

ATKINS LEMON MOUSSE

Prep time: 50 min

Servings: 8

Per Serving: Carbs: 3 g, Fat: 21 g, Protein: 9.4 g, Calories: 246

Ingredients

- 7 large whole eggs
- One 1 oz. package of unsweetened gelatin powder
- (unsweetened) ¼ cup lemon juice from freshly squeezed
- lemon 1 ½ fl. oz. orange liquor or brandy
- 6 individual packets of sucralose based sugar substitute
- 1 ½ cups heavy cream

Instructions

1. In a large bowl, mix gelatin in freshly squeezed lemon juice. Gently, place the bowl over a saucepan full of simmering water (make sure water doesn't touch the bottom of the bowl). Boil the eggs, peel them and separate the whites from the yolks; add the yolks to a saucepan and transfer the whites into a large bowl.
2. In a saucepan, whisk together the sugar substitute and the egg yolks. Keep cooking while stirring constantly over medium-high heat for about 4 minutes or until a candy thermometer indicates 180 degree F. Remove from heat; stir in orange liquor or brandy. Transfer to a large bowl.
3. Using an electric beater, beat egg whites for about 2 minutes. Meanwhile, in another large bowl, beat the heavy cream until firm peaks form. Add the egg whites into gelatin-yolk mixture and combine. Slowly, add the whipped cream. Check for sweetness; add more sugar substitute if necessary. Cover with aluminum foil and freeze until chilled. Enjoy!

YUMMILICIOUS GINGER FLAN

Prep time: 65 min

Servings: 6

Per Serving: Carbs: 3.5 g, Fat: 25 g, Protein: 4.7 g, Calories: 264

Ingredients

- 3 egg yolks (from large eggs)
- 2 large whole eggs
- 1 cup tap water
- 3 tsp. ginger
- 1 ½ cups heavy whipped cream
- 6 packets of sucralose based sugar sweetener
- 1 tsp. vanilla extract

Instructions

1. Pre-heat oven to 350°F. Fill a roasting pan half way with boiling water and place it on center shelf in the oven.
2. In a blender, add the whole eggs, egg yolks, tap water, whipped cream, vanilla extract, ginger and sugar substitute. Combine until smooth mixture is formed.
3. Use a sieve to pour the mixture into a 1-quart baking dish. Gently, place the dish in a roasting pan. Bake for about half an hour or until a knife put in the center comes out clean.
4. Remove and let it cool on a wire rack. Spray a plastic wrap sheet with a cooking spray, lay it directly over the baking dish and freeze it for about 3 hours in refrigerator.
5. Take away the plastic wrap and remove flan from the mold by placing a plate over the top and flipping it onto a table to make sure the pan is now upside down on the plate. Serve.5 Smoothies

SMOOTHIES

ATKINS COFFEE EGGNOG

Prep time: 5 min

Servings: 4

Per Serving: Carbs: 2.1 g, Fat: 25 g, Protein: 4.4 g, Calories: 308

Ingredients

- 1 tsp. sucralose based sugar substitute
- ½ tsp. vanilla extract
- 1 cup decaffeinated coffee
- 1 cup whipped heavy cream
- 3 fl. oz. rum (optional)
- 2 large whole eggs
- 1/8 tsp. ground cinnamon

Instructions

1. In a medium mixing bowl, beat the whole eggs and Sucralose sugar substitute. Add vanilla extract, whipped cream, coffee, and rum; combine well to form a smooth mixture.
2. Top with cinnamon and enjoy your coffee eggnog.

CREAMILICOUS STRAWBERRY SMOOTHIE

Prep time: 5 min

Servings: 2

Per Serving: Carbs: 5.6 g, Fat: 22 g, Protein: 26 g, Calories: 336

Ingredients

- 6 medium sized strawberries
- 2 servings strawberry based whey
- protein ½ cup heavy whipped cream
- 1 tsp. raw vanilla extract
- 2 cups tap water
- 2 packets sucralose based sugar sweetener

Instructions

1. In a blender, add strawberries, whey protein, whipped cream, tap water, vanilla and sucralose based sugar sweetener and blend until very smooth.

AVOCADO GAZPACHO SMOOTHIE

Prep time: 5 min

Servings: 1

Per Serving: Carbs: 4.7 g, Fat: 38 g, Protein: 9 g, Calories: 420

Ingredients

- 1 California avocado fruit without skin and seed
- 1 oz. soft goat cheese
- 2 tsp. freshly squeezed lime juice
- 1 tbsp. heavy whipped cream
- 2 tsp. chives, chopped
- 1/8 tsp. salt
- 1 cup tap water

Instructions

1. Place avocado in a blender. Add other ingredients and blend until a smooth mixture is formed. If required, you can also add extra water, 1 tbsp. at a time to reach desired consistency.
2. Pour the smoothie into the serving glass, and savor this exquisite blend with chives. Serve immediately.

ATKINS ALMOND RASPBERRY SMOOTHIE

Prep time: 5 min

Servings: 1

Per Serving: Carbs: 8.3 g, Fat: 15 g, Protein: 30.5 g, Calories: 300

Ingredients

- ¾ cup unsweetened original almond
- milk ½ cup raspberries
- 1 serving soy protein powder
- 20 each almonds

Instructions

1. In a blender, combine almond milk, protein powder, raspberries and almonds; pulse until smooth. You can also add 2 scoops of ice if desired.
2. Serve immediately.

~

TROPICAL RASPBERRY SMOOTHIE

Prep time: 5 min

Servings: 1

Per Serving: Carbs: 11.4 g, Fat: 30 g, Protein: 11.6 g, Calories: 357

Ingredients

- 4 oz. tofu, silken yet firm
- ½ cup coconut cream
- ½ cup raspberries (preferably red)
- 2 tsp. sucralose based sugar sweetener
- ¼ tsp. coconut extract
- 2-3 ice cubs (optional)

Instructions

1. In a blender, add coconut milk, tofu, red raspberries, coconut extract and sugar sweetener; blend until smooth.
2. With the blender already running, add ice cubes, one after the other, and blend until smooth.
3. Pour the smoothie into the serving glass, and top with raspberries and whipped cream, if desired. Serve immediately.

MY FINAL REQUEST...

Being a smaller author, reviews help me tremendously!

It would mean the world to me if you could leave a review by clicking the image below which will take you directly to the review section for this book.

Customer reviews

☆☆☆☆☆ 5 out of 5

12 customer ratings

5 star	▓▓▓▓▓▓▓▓▓▓	100%
4 star		0%
3 star		0%
2 star		0%
1 star		0%

˅ How does Amazon calculate star ratings?

Review this product

Share your thoughts with other customers

Write a customer review

If you liked reading this book and learned a thing or two, please click this link:

>> Click here to leave a brief review on Amazon. It

only takes 30 seconds but means so much to me!

Thank you and I can't wait to see your thoughts.

CONCLUSION

I hope this book has helped you learn everything that you need to know about losing weight successfully through the Atkins Diet program. All of details about how you can implement the program effectively have been covered. The information covered in this book should allow you to set proper expectations and prepare yourself for the challenges ahead. Keep in mind that if you follow the diet plan closely, you can lose weight and keep it off forever.

The next step is to get started. Weigh in. Decide on your weight goal. Get yourself a carb counter. Buy ketosis sticks. Create a chart for monitoring your progress. Write a shopping list. Plan your menu and always keep your eyes on the prize!

Thank you and good luck!

SPECIAL BONUS!

Want This Bonus book for FREE?

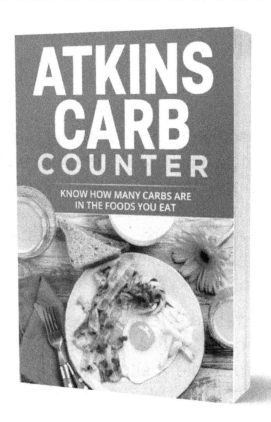

Get **FREE** unlimited access to it and all of my new books by joining the Fan Base!

CPSIA information can be obtained
at www.ICGtesting.com
Printed in the USA
BVHW010332080521
606756BV00008B/1785

9 781802 830422